the Sculpt plan

A Busy Woman's Flexible Guide *to*
Losing Weight, Feeling Great, *and*
Shifting Your Mindset *for* Life

Anita Rincón, M.S.

FAIR WINDS

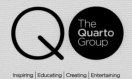

Brimming with creative inspiration, how-to projects, and useful information to enrich your everyday life, Quarto.com is a favorite destination for those pursuing their interests and passions.

© 2023 Quarto Publishing Group USA Inc.
Text © 2023 Sculpt Enterprises LLC
Photography © 2023 Quarto Publishing Group USA Inc.

First Published in 2023 by Fair Winds Press,
an imprint of The Quarto Group,
100 Cummings Center, Suite 265-D, Beverly, MA 01915, USA.
T (978) 282-9590 F (978) 283-2742 Quarto.com

Fair Winds Press titles are also available at discount for retail, wholesale, promotional, and bulk purchase. For details, contact the Special Sales Manager by email at specialsales@quarto.com or by mail at The Quarto Group, Attn: Special Sales Manager, 100 Cummings Center, Suite 265-D, Beverly, MA 01915, USA.

26 25 24 23 22   1 2 3 4 5

ISBN: 978-0-7603-7706-2

Digital edition published in 2023
eISBN: 978-0-7603-7707-9

Library of Congress Cataloging-in-Publication Data available

Design: Galbreath Design
Cover Image: Sculpt Enterprises LLC
Page Layout: Galbreath Design
Photography: Sculpt Enterprises LLC, Jessielyn Palumbo, and Shutterstock on pages 13, 18, 22, 27, 34, 36, 47, 55, 56, 80, 86, 95, 97, 101, and 111.

Printed in USA

DISCLAIMER The material in this book is for informational purposes only and not provided or intended as any form of medical consultation, evaluation, or treatment, or as substitute for the advice and care of your physician. As with all wellness, weight loss, or weight management efforts or regimens, you are advised to seek medical advice to make sure it is appropriate for your individual circumstances and to determine if any possible modification to the program contained in this book is required. If you have been diagnosed with any condition, please consult with your health care professional before beginning this or any other wellness, weight loss, or weight management program. The program is not intended for children. The author and the publisher expressly disclaim responsibility for any adverse effects that may result from the use or application of the information contained in this book.

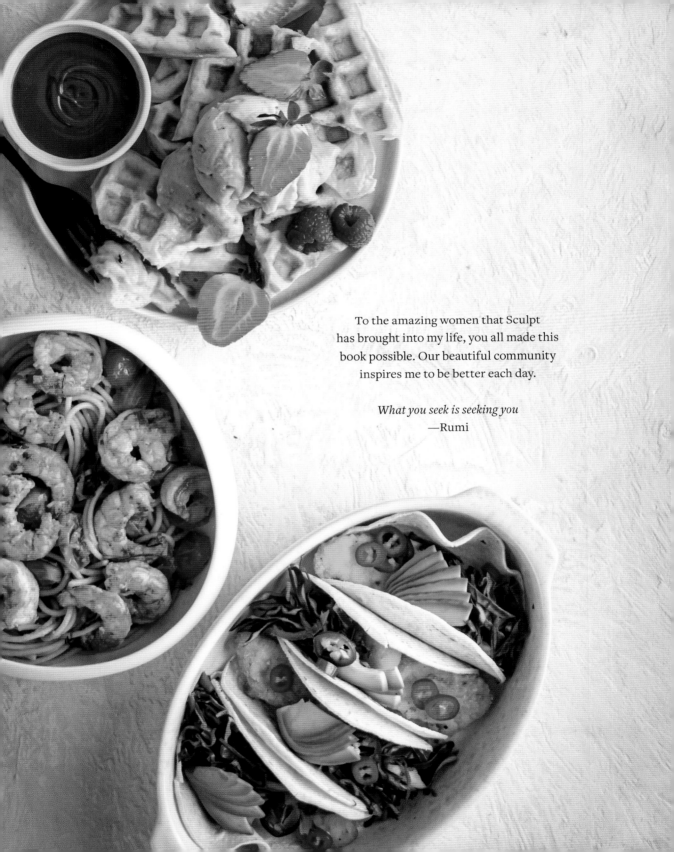

To the amazing women that Sculpt
has brought into my life, you all made this
book possible. Our beautiful community
inspires me to be better each day.

What you seek is seeking you
—Rumi

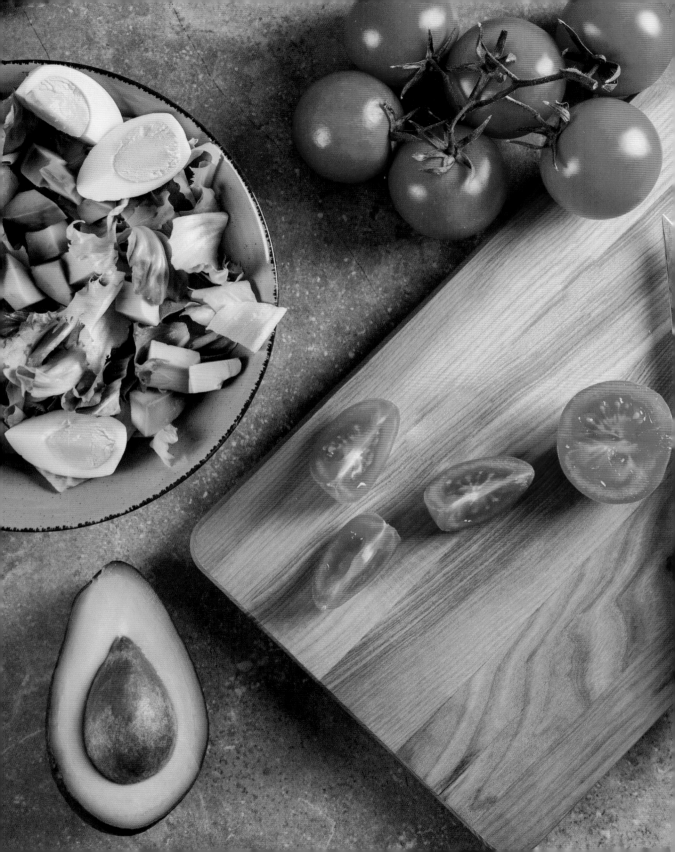

contents

introduction

"I NEED TO LOSE WEIGHT." Many of us have heard that voice inside a billion times. How often have we started yet another new diet, just to gain those same pounds back, plus more? And we're not alone. In 2018, the Centers for Disease Control and Prevention (CDC) reported that more than 56 percent of American women attempt to lose weight every year. But even with so many diets out there, overweight and obesity rates continue to skyrocket. The numbers are staggering: More than two out of three adult women in America are overweight or have obesity. Among Latina women, the number is three out of four. For Black women, it is four out of five.

Losing weight is hard enough, but the real challenge is maintaining weight loss without falling into old habits. It's no coincidence that only one in five adults who intentionally lost 10 percent or more of their body weight were able to maintain it for even a full year. There are thousands of diets dedicated to quick weight loss—but the one component that so many of them miss is how to create lasting success. Diets don't help us plan for life *after* the diet.

hi, i'm anita

To be honest with you, I was never the health or fitness-enthusiast type. But for as long as I can remember, I dieted on and off, seeking the happiness I was sure would come from hitting a certain weight or a certain size. I tried every diet out there, including cutting out entire food groups, like carbs or fat. I could usually get the weight off, but you can guess the problem: I simply couldn't keep it off.

Each diet became more restrictive than the last, as if I was the problem and I had to punish myself by tightening the rules even more. Not knowing any better, I assumed that was just the way weight loss had to be done. My weight fluctuated constantly. The more I dieted, the more weight I gained, and the more exhausted, lost, and frustrated I felt.

I finally got my wake-up call in 2017 after a series of life-changing events—moving to the United States from my native Finland, becoming an entrepreneur, and prioritizing my business over my health.

I'd gained 80 pounds (close to 40 kg). That's when reality hit. I was no longer just carrying a few extra pounds. In medical terms, my body mass index (BMI) now fell within the obesity range.

I remember feeling frustrated, embarrassed, and angry because I had lost control of my weight and my health somewhere along the way. I was twenty-nine years old and had been a serial dieter most of my life. How could I have managed to be structured and successful in many areas of my life, yet I couldn't get my weight under control?

Sound familiar? When I think back on this time, I wish I hadn't been so hard on myself. If only I'd known then what I know now! Weight gain rarely happens because of a single factor. An unhealthy lifestyle is the sum of little habits that slowly creep into our daily lives until they become a regular part of our routine. They're comfortable to us, and that makes them hard to break. If you feel like you're about to give up after all the times you've tried and failed to lose weight, then this book is for you.

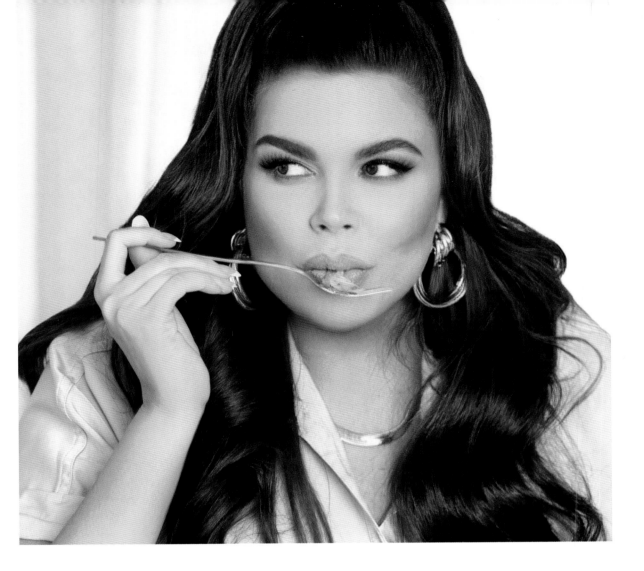

how sculpt was born

Let's rewind for a minute. When I was fresh out of college, I moved to New York City to start my first company, Rincón Cosmetics. It took off faster than I could have dreamed. I quickly got the opportunity to work with many well-known Hollywood makeup artists, celebrities, and nearly every trendsetter in the world of beauty. Within the first year, I was invited to give interviews and speak at events, and even offered my own TV show. My life was suddenly consumed by the whirlwind of work, work, and more work.

People often think the beauty world is all glitz and glam. In reality, I spent my days sitting in front of a computer from the moment I woke up through the late hours of the night. Like many young entrepreneurs, I didn't think I could afford to set boundaries between work and other parts of life. The company grew so quickly that I barely got to sleep at night and my days were consumed with stressing about the next deadline, quarterly sales goal, or product launch.

As you might expect, watching what I ate and making time to exercise were at the bottom of my to-do list. Scratch that—they weren't on my list at all. I had food delivered almost every day because I told myself I didn't have the time to cook or get groceries. And after a long and stressful day, I would often treat myself to unhealthy foods because hey, *I deserved it, right?* I couldn't make time to go to the gym because it would mean not finishing that day's workload. But I told myself that this was a normal part of running a business and that I would make up for it one day when I wasn't as busy. Of course, that "less busy" day never came.

I lived with that unhealthy mindset for two full years before stepping on that scale and getting a reality check. I was mostly in denial until that point; at five foot nine, I'm pretty tall and that disguised my weight gain to a degree. But my behavior had changed: I stopped shopping for new clothes, and I knew I wasn't happy with how I looked or the way I felt. I caught myself making excuses to skip gatherings or events. I didn't feel comfortable in my skin, and I didn't want others to see me like that.

And it wasn't just my appearance that I was unhappy with. I was getting sick all the time with strange symptoms the doctors couldn't make sense of. They'd prescribe antibiotics to take "just in case." I'd get intense migraines multiple times a week. My period cramps were off the charts. I tried to drop the weight with—you guessed it—dieting, but none of my old ways seemed to work anymore.

Convinced that there had to be a medical reason inhibiting my weight loss, I went to see one more doctor. I was prescribed yet another course of antibiotics along with the advice to try "eating less and exercising more." First I felt embarrassed, but that quickly turned to anger. I thought about the millions of women who are brushed off and made to feel bad with the suggestion that managing our weight would be a piece of cake if we just had a little self-control.

I'd had enough. I didn't know it then, but that doctor's visit marked a breaking point that changed my life forever. It was time to take a hard look at my priorities. Initially, I felt lost and unsure about how to make a change. All I knew was that I refused to feel like a prisoner in my own body any longer.

Rather than turning to the latest trending diet, I started fresh. I began researching the link between food, weight, and health, and that led to pursuing a formal education in nutrition. As young girls, we're taught to divide food into "good" and "bad," and many of us have been pushed from our earliest years to believe that healthy eating should feel like a punishment. I was ready to make a change and *unlearn* many of the things I'd considered part of a healthy lifestyle.

Let's face it, diets don't focus on learning about nutrition and how we can use it to our benefit. They've always been about losing weight in record time—often with shortcuts and feeling bad about ourselves through every step of the process. Ironically, demonizing certain foods and considering them off-limits often has the opposite effect, making us crave them even more. If someone tells you that you can't have pizza, then pizza is all you will be thinking about.

Little by little, I applied what I learned. The pounds began dropping, and I felt more energized and confident in my body each day. And just like that, the rest of the pieces of the puzzle fell into place. My migraines were less frequent, and my mystery symptoms disappeared. My periods became much more manageable. My skin was glowing, and my hair and nails were strong and shiny, a cherry on top that I hadn't expected. I was overjoyed to realize that simple food choices could change how I looked *and* how I felt.

I finally understood that to lose weight, I didn't have to feel bad about myself, succumb to a punishing diet or compulsive calorie counting. Every day I was getting closer to the version of myself that I wanted to become. By taking it meal by meal and pound by pound, I regained control of my weight and repaired the damage that dieting had done to my body and health over the years.

Soon, other people noticed the changes that were shining through. Everywhere I went, whether it was my office, the bank, or the supermarket, I was asked about the secret behind my weight loss. Yet how I did it was far from miraculous, and that made me realize just how many women like me were out there trying to navigate the conflicting information overload that practically swallows us when it comes to weight loss.

The *Sculpt* community was born out of the same passion that led me to start my beauty brand years before: To make women feel genuinely happy in their own skin. Only this time, I wanted it to mean permanent, lasting change.

Sculpt is about helping you transform your relationship with your body by taking control of your life and how you live it. I brought on dietitians, trainers, and experts in the psychology behind weight loss—the same extraordinary team that has been working tirelessly beside me for years to build evidence-based, female-focused weight management solutions that work. Together, we created an accessible lifestyle program to help every woman, of every size and age, reach the goals she has set out to achieve.

Sculpt is about finding joy in eating the food that you love and rediscovering movement in new ways, all while simplifying your already busy life. When it comes to weight loss, I will never tell you whether you should or shouldn't lose weight. Like any other decision over your body, it's a very personal one. It's no one else's place to tell you what to do with your body. I don't like to be told what to do, either! Plus, I wholeheartedly believe that you can be happy in your own skin at any size or weight as long as *you* are comfortable.

If you have made the decision that you want to lose weight, my role here is to guide you and set you up for success, no matter what the reasons are behind your choice to embark on this journey. Maybe you picked up this book because you feel unhappy at your current weight. Perhaps you feel like you're at your wit's end after committing to a bunch of diets that didn't work in the long run. I know from experience how frustrating it can be, and that's why I didn't think twice about the opportunity to share this book with you. I look at it as my responsibility to the community that's given me so much.

This program didn't take shape overnight, and you will learn in the pages to come that it goes well beyond weight loss. It started as my personal quest to change the way I *looked*, which then became about how I *felt*. It was—and continues to be—an ongoing evolution; the wave of positivity from my new lifestyle has seeped into every aspect of my life.

My changed relationship with food inspired me to go back to graduate school and pursue a master's degree in nutrition science with a specialization in obesity and weight management. Nutrition is an ever-developing science, and I unravel how you can make it work to your advantage with a simple set of principles. Over the years, I've spent thousands of hours researching women's health and weight management, followed by years of hands-on experience working with women like you—women who want to turn their lives around, not through shortcuts but with a complete lifestyle reset in simple, achievable steps. So, are you ready to begin? Let's go!

CHANGING YOUR LIFE

Don't worry, this isn't a book that leaves you with no real steps to take. To make a lasting change in your lifestyle, you must know that you deserve to live a healthy life and make caring for yourself a top priority. Not after you're 10, 20, or 50 pounds lighter, or when you fit into that old pair of jeans, but today, right now, and every day. If you use this book the way it's intended, your life can get better than you could have ever imagined—and don't be surprised if your weight is the least of it!

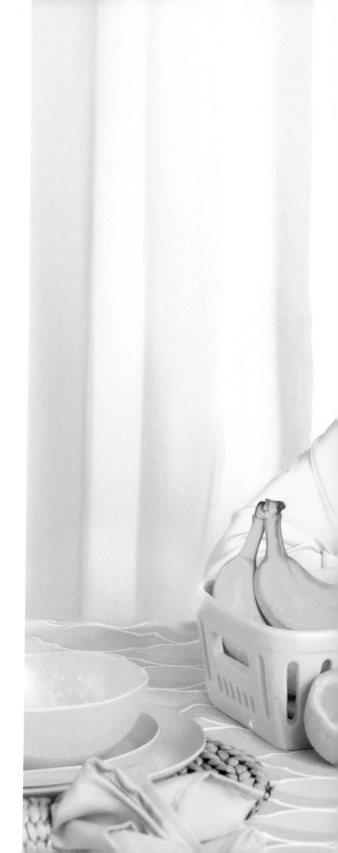

ready

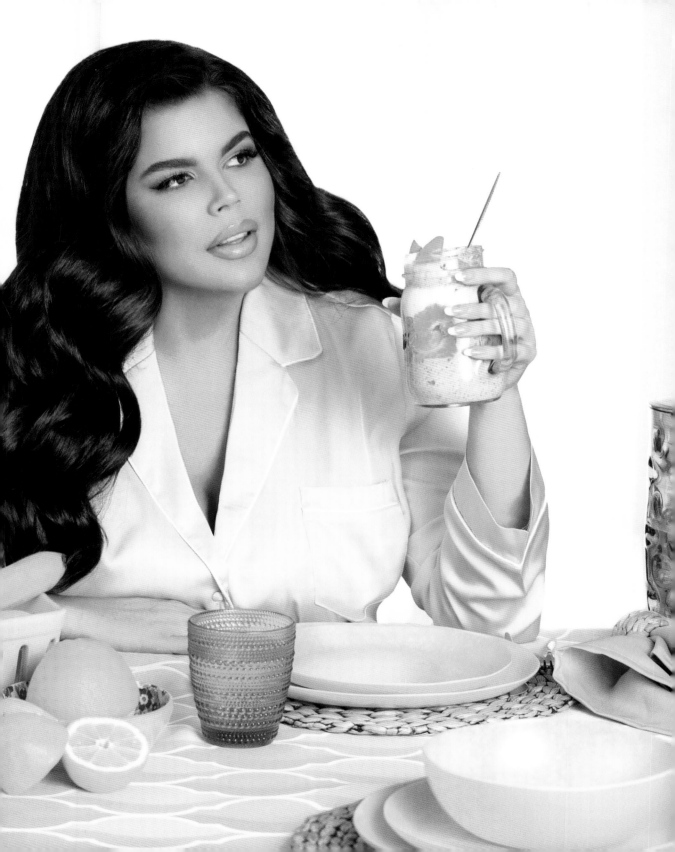

throwing out the rulebook

THE FACT THAT YOU'VE PICKED UP THIS BOOK means that something within you has shifted. You're ready to commit to living the healthier life you deserve. There is no better time to start than right now, and I am so proud of you for taking this step!

First things first: This isn't a diet book. It's about building a phenomenal life, one meal at a time. I wrote it because I want everyone to have access to a comprehensive program that covers every inch of the journey—one that goes much deeper than the average health book. And while this may sound like a big statement, it's one I can confidently make: If you follow it and embrace it as a lifestyle, it is the last program you will need.

I've made it my mission to provide a simple yet effective system for real women with real struggles, real jobs and careers, and real responsibilities. It's a program that adjusts even to the most hectic lifestyle and helps you take back power over your health. Spoiler alert: This means rebuilding a positive relationship with food, cultivating eating habits that benefit you, and enjoying what you eat. Ultimately, real success happens when we make the journey enjoyable. You're now officially part of a strong community of like-minded, inspiring women that welcomes you with open arms. For years, women who love *Sculpt* have been asking me for a lifestyle program to follow. With this book and its interactive parts, I'm finally able to deliver—directly to all of you. I hope you take full advantage of everything it offers as you aspire to more every day.

When we are in weight loss mode, we purposefully create an imbalance between energy intake and expenditure. That's a fancy way of saying that when the aim is to lose weight, we adjust the number of calories we eat to be less than the calories we burn. This is accurate and backed by decades of research. But this narrow view only considers two basic elements. We are not robots, and it's much more complex than that for most people.

When you put optimal nutrition and exercise habits into practice, you must also find a balance between work and rest, establish a routine to get high-quality sleep, and lean on your support system.

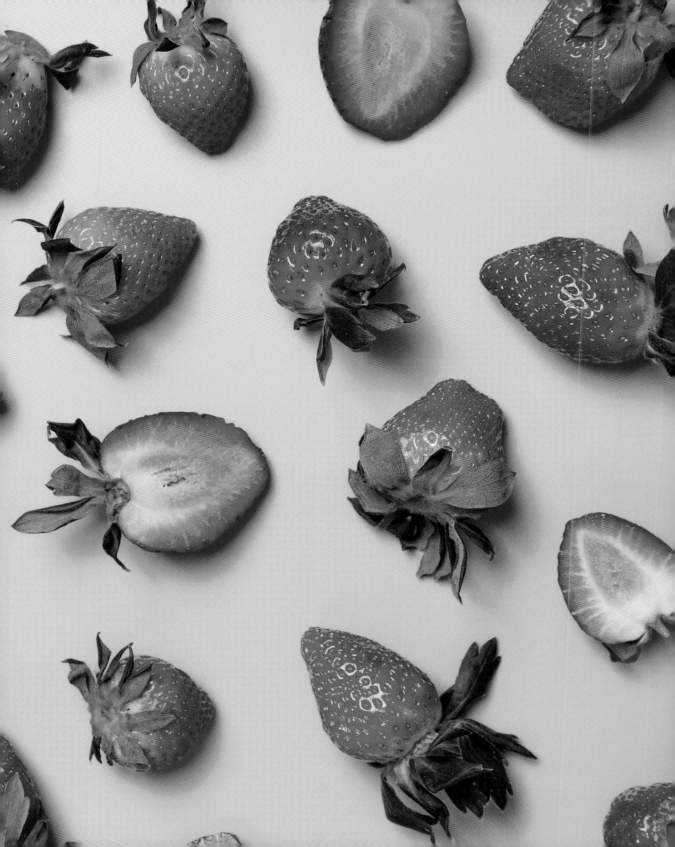

frequently asked questions

DO I NEED TO COUNT CALORIES?

No, you won't have to do any calorie counting! With the Meal Builder system in chapter 6, everything is adjusted for you. Just select the foods that you want to eat from each category, then build your meals and snacks around your personal preferences. No two people like the same foods, and no two plates should have to look the same, either.

DO I NEED TO BUY FANCY EQUIPMENT?

You can do perfectly fine without buying any expensive kitchen gadgets or workout equipment. I've listed my favorite kitchen essentials in chapter 2, along with suggestions for home workout gear in chapter 8.

WHAT IF I DON'T LIKE CERTAIN FOODS?

No worries, I got you! There's nothing more boring than lack of variety when it comes to eating. Your Meal Builder in chapter 6 lets you create your own meals by mixing and matching from different food groups. You get detailed instructions for putting together every meal, and there are hundreds of options to choose from with the help of the swap tables. Whether you enjoy all types of food, follow a gluten-free or dairy-free diet, or you are vegan or vegetarian, you'll always find meals that work for you.

WHEN WILL I SEE RESULTS?

Many factors will shape your individual rate of weight loss, such as your activity level and how your metabolism responds. If you stick to the program and work on building healthier habits every day, the only possible outcome is success! I've witnessed results varying from a steady 1 to 2 pounds (½ to 1 kg) a week to 5 pounds (2.5 kg) or more in the first week. Others are more likely to drop weight in crashes every couple of weeks.

Remember, every body is unique. I encourage you to give yours a chance to catch up as you progress through the program. Give it some time to get used to the new lifestyle changes!

HOW OFTEN SHOULD I EAT?

In this program, you're going to eat often! Each day includes five satisfying meals and snacks every three to four hours: breakfast, AM snack, lunch, PM snack, and dinner. You can switch your meals around according to your own schedule as long as you aim for your first meal to take place before 9 a.m. and the last meal before 10 p.m. Find the details for building meals in chapter 6.

HOW LONG DOES IT TAKE TO PREP MEALS FOR THE WEEK?

You can choose between two methods of meal prep: once a week or twice a week. This will depend mainly on the food and recipes that you've selected for the days ahead. I suggest choosing recipes based on your schedule for the week and how much time you'll have to spare in the kitchen. For more on meal prep and building your kitchen confidence, flip to chapter 7.

HOW MANY DAYS A WEEK WILL I WORK OUT?

For the fitness portion of this program, claim your access to the app with six interactive workouts a week (with home, gym, and minimal equipment options). You don't have to complete all six workouts as long as you're aiming to incorporate some form of movement each day—even if it's thirty minutes of walking divided into two or three mini walks. The important thing is to find an activity you enjoy! Check out chapter 8 for everything you need to know about exercise and staying active.

how it all started

You could say I was the program's very own guinea pig because I was the first to test every part of it. And there are many things that I wish someone had told me when I was starting my journey. It was trial and error, discovering what worked, what didn't, and what created lasting results. I journaled every detail and kept track of my daily progress. We've combined my own experiences and the expertise of professionals I have the pleasure of working with today. The result is this complete lifestyle program—one that can be tailored to meet every woman's individual goals.

I've learned that when people hold back from pursuing the things they want in life, it's usually because they're scared that they won't succeed. If that describes you, I can assure you right now that you won't need to be perfect on this journey. You don't need to be an expert in the kitchen or even passionate about working out. I will give you the tools to succeed, and all I need from you is to show up consistently every day, put those tools to use, and trust the process.

HERE TO TRANSFORM YOUR LIFE

Sculpt doesn't call for luxurious or expensive ingredients to cook your meals. In fact, you can make your meals as simple or elaborate as you want. We need our meals to fit our hectic schedules—not the other way around. My style of eating is all about assembling meals with what I have available: simple, delicious cooking with easy-to-find ingredients that you can use on repeat whenever you feel like it. Food should always taste good, but I don't like to toil away over the stove making complex recipes that require tons of ingredients or hours of prep.

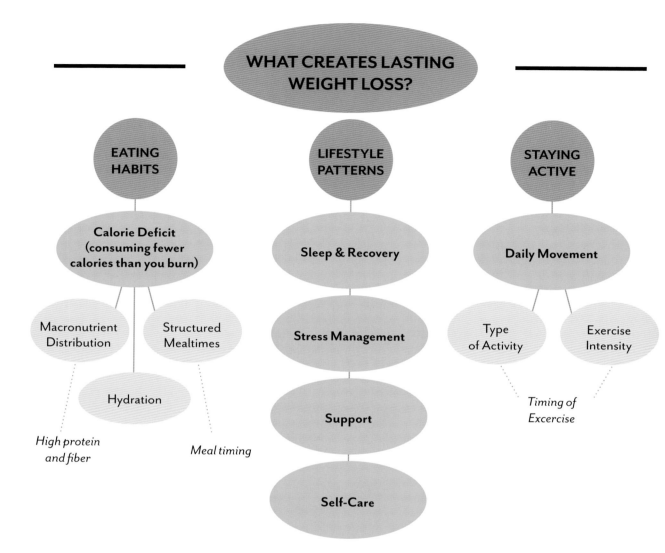

WHAT CREATES LASTING WEIGHT LOSS?

EATING HABITS

Calorie Deficit (consuming fewer calories than you burn)

Macronutrient Distribution

Structured Mealtimes

Hydration

High protein and fiber

Meal timing

LIFESTYLE PATTERNS

Sleep & Recovery

Stress Management

Support

Self-Care

STAYING ACTIVE

Daily Movement

Type of Activity

Exercise Intensity

Timing of Excercise

Meal prep is the answer to having timesaving, make-ahead meals at your fingertips. It's what will allow you to keep living your life to the fullest while still hitting your health goals. Whether you prepare your meals once or twice weekly, I'll help you stay organized and structured with just one trip to the grocery store a week. Prepping your own meals also minimizes those hidden additives and preservatives that go into ultra-processed food. Your mind will be clearer, making you more productive and helping you get more out of your days. Win-win!

You'll never have to feel like you can't progress toward your goals because of lack of time. I'll share the guidelines, and you choose the flavors you love within them. In chapter 7, I'll show you what to stock in your pantry, fridge, and freezer with a ready-made list of essentials and meal prep instructions. Plus, you'll find all my staples for meal inspiration in the recipe section, starting on page 112. You'll never have to leave a meal to guesswork again.

FALL IN LOVE WITH MOVEMENT

While weight loss starts in the kitchen, staying active plays an important role in achieving the results you desire. Movement is an essential component of a healthy, balanced, less stressed life. Even if you only have limited time to work out or no access to a gym, no need to worry.

I used to absolutely dread the gym and the mere thought of working out until I realized that enjoyable exercise doesn't mean the same thing for everyone. Some of us like high-impact workouts in a gym setting, while others prefer to exercise at home or outdoors. It comes down to trying different things, finding what suits you best, and then sticking to it—and that won't be nearly as hard when you enjoy it!

Over time, exercising has become a therapeutic necessity to me. I look at cooking my weekly meals as self-care time that's dedicated solely to my own well-being and health.

The bottom line is that your weight loss journey shouldn't be miserable in any way. This program aims to transform what you may have once dreaded into something that you look forward to. That's where the magic happens, and it becomes a lifelong habit.

the program at a glance: ready, set, thrive!

The *Sculpt* program has three phases. The Ready phase helps you take a closer look at the reasons behind weight gain, and it identifies the unhealthy habits that have been holding you back. You'll start getting ready for the program with activities like goal setting, creating healthier routines that will benefit your journey, and learning how to track your progress accurately.

In the Set phase, you'll learn how to assemble your meals and add enjoyable movement to your daily life, while continuing to apply all the tools gained in the Ready phase to help you reach your goal weight. This is the center of the program—one that combines flexible meal ideas with an exercise program that you can fit in even on the busiest days. I'll answer all your questions and provide clear guidance no matter what stage of the journey you are in.

And I won't leave you hanging once you've successfully met your desired weight goal. Transitioning to the Thrive phase helps you ease out of weight loss mode by making strategic, small changes to your eating. At the same time, you'll continue sticking to the lifestyle changes made in the Ready stage. This way, we'll ensure that a rebound effect doesn't occur and undo all your hard work.

In the chapters that follow, you'll learn all about the program. We'll start with the importance of shifting your mindset and rethinking your relationship with food. The best part of the program is that all this can be achieved:

- without "magic" diets
- without deprivation
- without compromises
- without boring meals
- without overcomplicating things

And remember, this is your journey, so make this book your own by taking notes, bookmarking, highlighting, marking pages with post-its, or screenshotting. Get excited! It's time to work!

your journey starts now

NOW WE'RE OFF TO THE FUN PART! Use this chapter to start the program, then revisit it to review the guidelines when you need to.

STEP 1:
lay the groundwork

Changing your lifestyle starts with a clear understanding of where you want to go and how you can get there. I don't believe in programs that dictate a rigid meal guide and expect you to follow it blindly. In chapter 3, we look at the counterproductive behaviors behind weight gain and replace those patterns with beneficial ones that will get you closer to your goals. In chapter 4, we set achievable goals and learn methods to track your progress accurately. Knowledge is power, and in chapter 5 we'll look at how the right nutrition can produce the results you desire and help you make the shift toward smarter food choices.

STEP 2:
find your group

You'll begin the program by identifying your current group based on how much weight you want to lose.

GROUP 1: 1-19 pounds (1-9 kg) to lose

GROUP 2: 20-39 pounds (10-19 kg) to lose

GROUP 3: 40-60 pounds (20-30 kg) to lose

If you want to lose more than 60 pounds (30 kg), for every additional 20 pounds (10 kg) you'll pick one item from the list of add-ons in chapter 6. This chapter explains the portion system in detail, giving you flexible instructions to make your meals work around your life.

Choosing a goal weight is fully up to you. Use the table on the next page for additional guidance, if needed. The height-to-weight ratio can help you find a healthy weight for your height based on the range determined by the CDC. It's there to help you ensure that the goal you set isn't under the recommended

find your group

Height	Recommended healthy weight range lbs (kg)		Group 1 lbs (kg)		Group 2 lbs (kg)		Group 3 lbs (kg)	
	from	*to*	*from*	*to*	*from*	*to*	*from*	*to*
4'10" (147 cm)	89 (40)	119 (54)	120 (55)	138 (63)	139 (64)	158 (73)	159 (74)	179 (84)*
4'11" (150 cm)	92 (42)	123 (55)	124 (56)	142 (64)	143 (65)	162 (74)	163 (75)	183 (85)*
5' (152 cm)	95 (43)	127 (58)	128 (59)	146 (67)	147 (68)	166 (77)	167 (78)	187 (88)*
5'1" (155 cm)	98 (45)	132 (60)	133 (61)	151 (69)	152 (70)	171 (79)	172 (80)	192 (90)*
5'2" (158 cm)	101 (46)	136 (62)	137 (63)	155 (71)	156 (72)	175 (81)	176 (82)	196 (92)*
5'3" (160 cm)	105 (48)	140 (63)	141 (64)	159 (72)	160 (73)	179 (82)	180 (83)	200 (93)*
5'4" (163 cm)	108 (49)	145 (66)	146 (67)	164 (75)	165 (76)	184 (85)	185 (86)	205 (96)*
5'5" (165 cm)	111 (50)	149 (68)	150 (69)	168 (77)	169 (78)	188 (87)	189 (88)	209 (98)*
5'6" (168 cm)	115 (52)	154 (70)	155 (71)	173 (79)	174 (80)	193 (89)	194 (90)	214 (100)*
5'7" (170 cm)	118 (54)	159 (72)	160 (73)	178 (81)	179 (82)	198 (91)	199 (92)	219 (102)*
5'8" (173 cm)	122 (55)	164 (74)	165 (75)	183 (83)	184 (84)	203 (93)	204 (94)	224 (104)*
5'9" (175 cm)	125 (57)	168 (76)	169 (77)	187 (85)	188 (86)	207 (95)	208 (96)	228 (106)*
5'10" (178 cm)	129 (59)	173 (78)	174 (79)	192 (87)	193 (88)	212 (97)	213 (98)	233 (108)*
5'11" (180 cm)	133 (60)	178 (81)	179 (82)	197 (90)	198 (91)	217 (100)	218 (101)	238 (111)*
6' (183 cm)	137 (62)	183 (83)	184 (84)	202 (92)	203 (93)	222 (102)	223 (103)	243 (113)*

*For every additional 20 pounds (10 kg), start in Group 3 and incorporate an add-on from the list in chapter 6.

healthy weight. Ultimately, your goal weight is as unique as you are, and you should set it to please yourself. We'll also be using other parameters to measure your progress. See chapter 4 for more on those metrics.

Keep in mind that your group at the beginning of your journey won't be your forever group. You will switch between groups as you lose weight during the program. If you start in group 3, you'll gradually switch to group 2 and then group 1 until you reach your goal weight. We'll talk about this in detail in chapter 6.

STEP 3:
locate your meal builder

Once you've identified your group, look for the Meal Builder in chapter 6. With *Sculpt*, you will eat five times a day, every three to four hours, starting with breakfast by 9 a.m. within thirty minutes of rising. Your last meal of the day should take place before 10 p.m.

Don't skip meals, especially breakfast! Skipping meals can lead to blood sugar spikes, often causing us to overeat by the time we get to the next meal. Plus, when we're starving and our blood sugar has dropped, we tend to grab whatever we can get our hands on—whether that's an actual meal or a handful of candy. Skipping meals negatively impacts our ability to focus and make decisions, too. Granted, it may not always be possible to eat every few hours—if you must skip a meal, see chapter 6.

The amount of weight you want to lose will influence the size of your portions: The higher your group number is, the larger your meals are. That's because the higher the body weight, the more calories the body burns at rest. As you get closer to your goal weight and switch to a lower group, the size of your meals becomes slightly smaller.

With the Meal Builder system, you'll find strategic guidelines for assembling your meals along with examples to fit five dietary variations: Standard, gluten-free, dairy-free, vegetarian, and vegan.

STEP 4:
get creative in the kitchen

Experiment with new flavors, spices, and fresh herbs to give your favorite foods a kick as you build your cooking confidence. Give mealtimes more variety by using the food swap tables starting on page 64. Whether you're looking for more options for proteins, starches, fats, veggies, or fruit, the swap function makes it easy to tailor your meals.

Be sure to have a stash of your favorite food staples and go-to ingredients. And always keep vegetables on hand—preferably fresh, but frozen and canned are great for convenience. For fruit, fresh or frozen is the way to go! Even when you're short on time, you'll always have options to choose from.

Starting on page 112, get inspired by big-flavor recipes! You can use your Meal Builder to come up with virtually any meal based on what you feel like eating. I've included some of my favorite staples to make your weeknights even easier. From all-American cooking to Mexican, Caribbean, Italian, or Chinese food, you'll find recipes inspired by different cultures, flavors, and cooking styles. Challenge yourself to try new foods and expand your horizons in the kitchen because you will love making all these dishes, whatever your cooking abilities are!

There are recipes for when you want to step up your cooking—for date nights or dinner parties with friends. You'll also find sweet treats to satisfy cravings. Each recipe's ingredient list is marked to identify the group they belong to, their suitability for any dietary restrictions or preferences you may have, and the time and level of effort the recipe requires.

STEP 5:
access your workouts

With the purchase of this book, you get three months of free access to the *Sculpt* fitness program through the app by entering thesculptplan.com/book. It's designed to complement your meals through an effective, fat-burning training combination. The workouts in the app maximize the time you spend exercising, meaning you burn calories during *and* after working out.

The exercise portion of the program is just as customizable as your meals! You'll have three options to choose from: Minimal equipment, home, and gym. There are workouts for fitness levels ranging from beginner to advanced, and they are built for your success by *Sculpt* trainers who specialize in female body transformations. You get access to six workouts per week—a combination of sculpting sessions, metabolic training, weight training, and cardio, as well as on-demand content, such as yoga and meditation to manage stress and improve your sleep.

Pick your workouts as your schedule allows, and exercise on your own terms when it's convenient for you. I highly recommend completing at least three sessions per week. Not feeling ready to commit to a full fitness program just yet? We'll go into more detail about movement and the variety of options for every level in chapter 8!

STEP 6:
meet your sculpt squad

This program goes beyond the book! We're with you every step of the way, virtually. You'll have access to your interactive workouts through the app, and it allows you to stay accountable with check-ins every two weeks. Even better, you get rewarded with actual prizes, like kitchen essentials and workout gear, for completing your check-ins regularly! Start by visiting the website to take advantage of all the extra features.

STEP 7:
road to a lifestyle

Sculpt is a lifestyle with a forever approach. A key part of the program starts *after* you've met your weight loss goal when you enter the Thrive phase. The ultimate

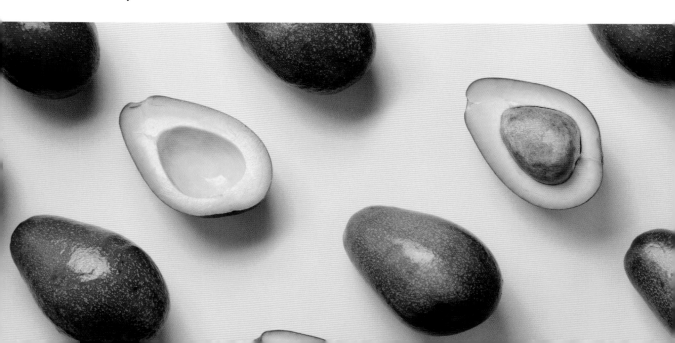

goal is to stick to the habits you learn as we make small adjustments to your meals until you reach your individual maintenance level. We'll talk about this transition in more detail in chapter 10.

the must haves

From here on out, we will be doing a lot of cooking at home. These are your must-have kitchen essentials to get started:

KITCHEN SCALE

A scale makes all the difference in cooking and food prep! Studies have shown that most of us underestimate how much we eat—by many estimates, between 30 and 46 percent. Over time, those extra calories can add up and produce weight gain. A kitchen scale is inexpensive and super simple to use; it will be your go-to tool as you get familiar with the program's portion sizes. The idea isn't to keep weighing your food forever, but a scale gives you a better understanding of how much food is going on your plate and helps you check on portion sizes whenever you feel unsure.

BLENDER

When you've only got minutes to put together a meal or snack, smoothies come through! They make a quick and nutritious breakfast. If you're a smoothie lover like me, a good blender will be one of your most frequently used kitchen tools. For single servings, I recommend choosing a compact bullet model to blend individual-sized smoothies, sauces, and dips. It can even be used in place of a food processor.

NONSTICK SKILLET

I love a nonstick skillet because it allows me to cook with little to no oil when I want to use my healthy fat portions on something else. Nonstick pans, whether traditional, ceramic-coated, or stainless steel, will be your best friend in healthy cooking. When picking a skillet, choose a large size that will allow you to cook bigger batches on your meal prep days.

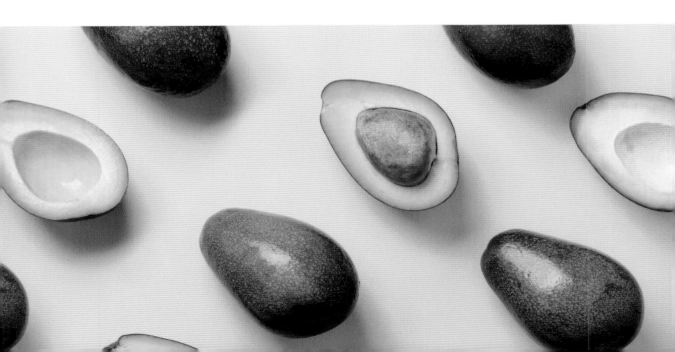

MEAL PREP CONTAINERS

For fridge storage and reheating purposes, I always go with leak-proof glass, stainless steel, or silicone containers. Glass is the safest option for the oven and microwave. Avoid heating food and drinks in plastic containers; it can cause chemicals in plastic to contaminate your food! If you go with a material other than glass or stainless steel for meal prep, silicone is your best bet. I use reusable silicone sandwich bags and freezer-friendly containers. Glass can be heavy and break; I usually choose silicone or stainless steel containers for meals on the go.

If you already have plastic containers, make sure they're BPA-free. Those are a much safer option to use, and they're environmentally friendly, too.

MEASURING TOOLS

When exploring new foods and cooking styles, precise measuring is essential. You probably have measuring cups in your kitchen already. If you're looking to upgrade, I recommend going with any set that comes with the basic sizes: teaspoon, tablespoon, ¼ cup, ⅓ cup, ½ cup, and 1 cup (or 1 dl).

CUTTING BOARDS

This may be an obvious one, but there's always room for improvement! I prefer plastic cutting boards; they're hassle-free and easy to clean. Wooden cutting boards absorb meat juices and harbor bacteria, plus you can't wash them in a dishwasher. If you have a wooden one, only use it for non-meat items. I recommend getting at least two cutting boards: One for proteins, including raw meats, and one for everything else.

the big question: at what rate can i expect to lose weight?

I know it's hard to wait when you want results. Your rate of weight loss is individual and will depend on the current state of your metabolism, the number of diets you've pursued in the past, the calorie intake your body was used to before starting the program, and your activity level—just to name a few factors. I've witnessed unbelievable results in women of all ages, whether they experience a drastic drop of 10 or more pounds (5 kg) in the beginning, a steady 1 to 2 pounds (½ to 1 kg) a week, or shed weight in periodic crashes. Generally people with more weight to lose will lose more weight initially, but that's not always the case.

My goal was to lose 80 pounds—although I ended up losing more than 100—but when I started, it took several weeks for the pounds to start shedding. I was convinced something was wrong with me. The number on the scale just wouldn't budge, so there had to be something strange going on in my body!

I stuck to the plan and trusted it wholeheartedly—and boom! Suddenly I lost 5 pounds (2½ kg). Another 5 pounds the week after. And yet another 5 pounds, followed by a steady 2 pounds (1 kg) a week. All I needed to do was allow my body to adjust to the new lifestyle changes. By doing that, I gave my slowed-down metabolism a chance to heal from all the excessive yo-yo dieting I'd put it through over the years. Your body is incredible and unique, and it's important to remember that whatever the rate of weight loss may look like for you.

COMMON FACTORS BEHIND YOUR RATE OF WEIGHT LOSS

Some common factors that can influence how quickly you lose weight include:

Consistency

In weight loss, consistency beats perfection. Think about consistency as your superpower: Showing up every day, even on those days when you don't feel like it, and putting your new habits to practice equals huge changes in the long term. So, if you put in 100 percent of your effort, you can count on getting 100 percent results out of it.

Genetics

Science is continually evolving, but what we know so far about the role that genetics play in our body weight is this: About 50 percent is determined by genetics and 50 percent is determined by our lifestyle choices, including eating habits and physical activity. While we can't do much about our genes, we have control over our eating and activity patterns, and that's what *Sculpt* focuses on.

Exercise

It's a no-brainer that the amount of exercise you incorporate in your program will have a positive effect on your results. But if you're not used to regular exercise, adding it to your routine can have a surprising effect in the beginning. You may see your weight stall or even go up a bit as your body responds to the new regimen. If you experience this, trust that it is just a temporary part of the process. Your body just needs some time to adjust. In the meantime, enjoy the non-scale benefits of movement, like better sleep, productivity, mood, and more energy!

don't feel frustrated!

It took a while for you to gain weight, and it wouldn't be realistic to lose it overnight. Be kind to yourself, patient with your body, and trust the process!

Hormones

Did you know that most women—some estimates go as high as 80 percent—suffer from a hormonal imbalance at some point in their lives? Because hormones can play an important role in weight loss, it's important to get your levels tested as part of your yearly blood work. This is often included in your annual checkup with a primary care provider, but I encourage you to ask if you don't think you've had it done before. Prioritize your annual checkups to learn about any potential underlying conditions that could affect your health.

Sleep

Did you know that continuous poor sleep can reduce, or even ruin your results? It's true. Studies have found that lack of sleep significantly hinders the rate of fat loss. When you're tired the next day, your brain's reward centers look for comfort causing the sleep-deprived brain to have trouble saying no to overeating and junk food. It's no surprise that poor sleep can lead to poor decision-making. So, for optimal results, a solid seven to nine hours of sleep per night is a must! We'll talk about creating a better bedtime routine for quality sleep in chapter 9.

taking back your life

THERE'S A REASON YOU'VE BEEN FEELING STUCK and out of control with your eating. It's because in real life, losing weight is much more complex than calories in, calories out. If it were that simple, everyone could do it!

Food is your body's fuel; it should make you feel good on the inside and out. Yet our eating often becomes a response to our emotions or external influences. In this chapter, we will focus on your eating patterns and making productive mindset shifts to:

- understand what drives your eating
- identify what's been keeping you from losing weight
- regain control over your eating
- build a positive relationship with food
- shift your habits for lasting success

Healthy eating habits come from having the tools to make good decisions and developing a positive relationship with food. By dismantling unhelpful thoughts and replacing them with a mindset that takes you closer to becoming your best version, you're building a strong foundation for lasting change. You got this!

the diet trap

Restrictive dieting just doesn't work for long-lasting results, no matter how dedicated we are to it. The senseless part is that we have been taught that we're the ones failing. We're told it's our lack of willpower that keeps us from shedding the excess weight we want to lose. In reality, it's not about willpower. Diets simply don't work because they are a temporary fix, with a start and an end date.

But these quick, restrictive diets have become all we know, whether its juice cleanses or extreme carb restriction, you name it, and they often have little to do with health. They consist of lists of foods we can't eat, teaching us to hate and fear food. That pursuit of perfection actually *prevents* us from working toward a healthier, more balanced lifestyle.

Let's be clear: Good choices do matter. We need to be mindful of portion sizes and recognize that eating oversized quantities of certain foods can sabotage our results. And it's important to understand why selecting some foods over others is more beneficial when the goal is to lose weight. But that's not the same as punishing ourselves with self-blaming thoughts when things don't go according to plan. Not only does that make us feel lousy and enjoy food less, but eventually, the vicious cycle of shame drives us to eat even more of

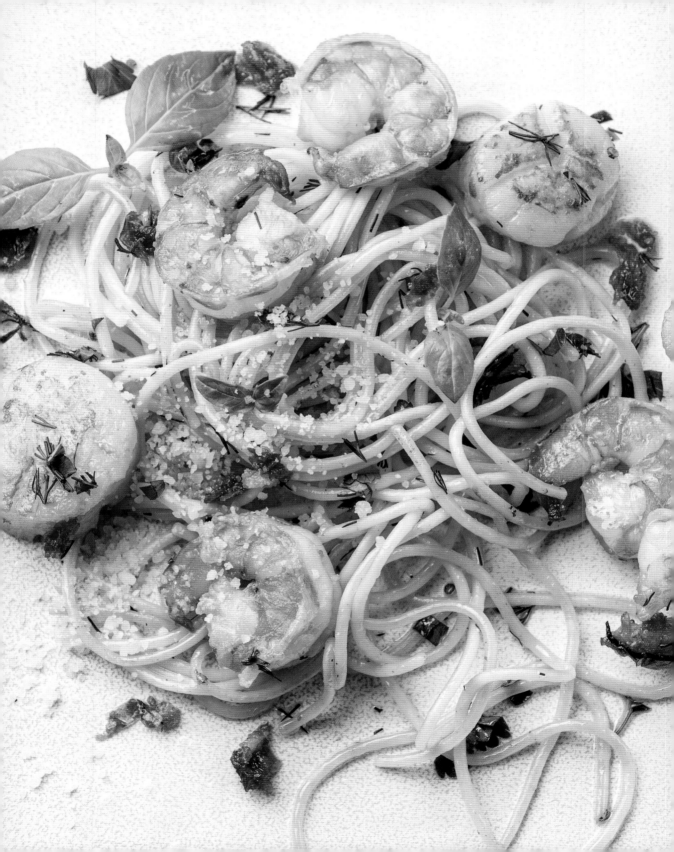

those "forbidden" foods to feel better. Sure, restrictive eating may work for a period of time, but eventually, we grow tired of it and return to our old ways.

Understanding what rooted habits have been preventing you from reaching your goals is the first step toward freeing yourself from them. Changing behavior requires acknowledging your thoughts and actions. By making a conscious switch to better outlets, you'll be laying the groundwork to prevent those old, unhealthy patterns from being repeated.

opening your mind

Healing my relationship with food and exercise was by far the most life-changing part of my journey. Just like having a dry mouth tells you to drink water, and heavy eyes tell you it's time to sleep, your body knows what foods and how much of them you need; it's programmed in you. But somewhere along the line, most of us stopped listening to our bodies' internal hunger and fullness cues. Instead, many of our choices are determined by our environment.

Luckily, it's never too late to unlearn. I should know—I had so many preconceptions around food that needed dismantling. Years of dieting had instilled in me that nutrition had to be categorized into two groups: Foods that were prohibited, which could only be made up for with a skipped meal or extra long workout, and approved diet foods I could eat without feeling bad afterward. And guess what that miserable mindset usually led to? Anything but losing weight!

Frankly, all that black-and-white thinking does is keep you from balance and moderation—two pillars of healthful eating. Today, I know how to identify and overcome sabotaging thought processes when they threaten to pull me back to my old ways. Developing a positive relationship with food and maintaining a healthy weight is all about finding pleasure in eating. And that doesn't mean indulging every day or sitting at home eating junk. It's about rediscovering the joy of eating.

In this book, we focus on progress, not perfection. Self-reflection and awareness of your feelings and behaviors are the key to creating positive change. If you can acknowledge that any real journey has ups and downs, it will help you be kinder to yourself along the way. There may be days when you don't stick to your meals or you skip a workout. You may feel unmotivated and not want to get out of bed. There may also be days when your scale doesn't seem to reflect your hard work. Those things are a perfectly normal part of any journey to long-term success.

DIVING DEEPER INTO LEARNED HABITS

Let's start by identifying repetitive behaviors in your life that have contributed to gaining weight. Often, habits are so ingrained in our daily lives that we hardly notice them. For instance, when you leave your home, you lock the door. Is there a thought process involved between you exiting and locking the door? Probably not. Same goes for brushing your teeth in the morning or drying off with a towel after showering.

celebrate small steps

It's easy to get excited about visible progress, but most of the time the real work is in the unquantifiable: The dismantling of unhelpful habits and the building of better ones. And when something isn't directly measurable, we often forget to celebrate it. Take the time to congratulate yourself on the small habits you're working on building every day!

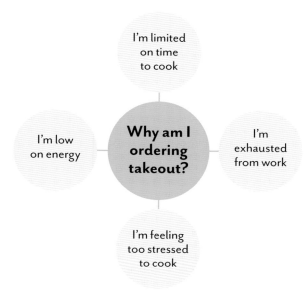

I'm limited on time to cook

I'm low on energy

Why am I ordering takeout?

I'm exhausted from work

I'm feeling too stressed to cook

With eating, habits can mean automatically turning to comfort food when you're sad, or grabbing a bag of chips as you tune into your favorite TV show. As natural as these things may feel now, you learned them all at some point. By repeating them day after day, they became a part of your routine. This goes for each habit you have, and some of them aren't doing you any good.

The first step to unlearning habits that are inhibiting your progress is identifying where they come from and what challenges and thoughts produce them. Once you are aware of how your habits developed, it's much easier to overcome them and avoid new unhelpful ones from forming! Similarly, replacing negative thinking with kind thoughts helps rebuild a positive sense of direction. Through consistency, you will transform your body and your mindset.

To give you an example, one of the main factors I can identify as a contributor to my weight gain was a habit of ordering takeout more times a week than I'd like to admit. In one study, 92 percent of American restaurant takeout meals were shown to contain excessive calories, posing a greater risk of excess weight for those who regularly consume them. It's easy to make the connection between frequent take-out meals and weight gain. But if you asked me back then, I would have told you I was limited on time, low on energy, exhausted from work, and too stressed out to cook, so I had no other choice but to depend on restaurant food.

To understand this habit on a deeper level, I should look into the thoughts that ran through my mind before grabbing my phone and placing an order. It wasn't always about lack of time. Some-times, I had the urge to order because takeout was a way to reward myself for a productive workday. Other times, I relied on it as a pick-me-up after a bad day. Or, if my partner ordered food to watch football with his friends, why shouldn't I? Maybe I couldn't fight the temptation because the food from that specific restaurant was just so delicious.

I'd justify it by telling myself that I would start a new, healthy life the next day. And that never hap-pened because the next day I would just repeat the same habit. Why? Because I wasn't seeing it as a factor in my weight gain, so I didn't plan to have smarter meal options available by the time I got home from work. In my mind, I simply believed that I didn't have a choice. And by doing nothing to change it, I was unconsciously allowing the habit to become part of my everyday routine.

examples to get you started

Struggle

Feeling exhausted	Not having enough time
Having low energy	Temptation
A stressful day at work	Peer pressure
Eating in social situations	Feeling sad

Thought

My friends will be offended if I don't eat this.

I'll just go to the gym tomorrow.

I can't be bothered to cook food.

I can't say no.

Cooking is too much work right now.

I deserve it as a reward.

Everyone else can have it, why can't I?

I just can't resist the temptation.

This will make me feel better.

Habit

Overeating	Late-night snacking
Emotional eating	Distracted or mindless eating
Skipping workouts	Uncontrollable eating
Snacking by the desk at work	Ordering delivery or takeout

Identifying Your Challenges

It's easier to put a plan in place when you know your triggers. Write down the personal struggles, thoughts, and habits that you can identify as your personal contributors to weight gain.

My struggle with _____ makes me think about _____. This leads to the habit of _____.

BREAKING IT DOWN

Once you understand how habits are formed, you can get ahead of the game by paying attention and identifying them whenever they occur. In my years of helping women on their individual journeys, I have learned that many of us share the same five struggles with weight loss.

- We take an all-or-nothing approach that causes us to abandon our goals when things don't go our way

- We prioritize other things over our health and can't find time to put ourselves first

- We experience confusion over what to eat and how much to eat to be healthy

- We have negative thoughts around food that control our eating

- We fall back into old habits after losing weight

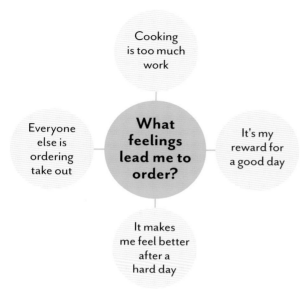

Cooking is too much work

Everyone else is ordering take out

What feelings lead me to order?

It's my reward for a good day

It makes me feel better after a hard day

rebuilding your mindset

The way we speak to ourselves is important, yet we rarely pay active attention to it. An all-or-nothing mindset can easily convince you of negative, false scenarios that can hamper your progress. And it's far from being your fault—all the misinformation that we have easy access to twenty-four hours a day creates so much unnecessary fear and confusion. In reality, your toughest obstacles live in your own mind.

The good news is that you can identify these thoughts and overcome them. Your brain is wired to love repetition and consistency—it's one reason those distorted thoughts are so successful! Luckily, the reverse is also true. The more you push positive thoughts forward by reframing negative thoughts, the easier it becomes to change your beliefs around them.

What are some negative thoughts you can recall telling yourself often? Write them down, along with a positive and more realistic replacement for each thought. Feeling stuck? Think about the common experiences listed in the sidebar on the previous page.

riding the wave

Most of us have a sweet tooth for something, whether it's comfort foods, candy, or salty snacks. To enjoy the food you love in a way that won't interfere with your progress, conquer your cravings with healthier swaps that are just as delicious. That's what the *Sculpt* meals are all about—enjoying food every day. Allowing yourself to indulge is important, and I'm not talking about some watered-down, light version of good food. You can make virtually any dish fit your Meal Builder! Watch as your cravings fade away when amazing food becomes part of your everyday life. Get inspired by new ways of making all your favorites in the recipe section starting on page 112.

breaking the cycle

Keep reframing your thoughts consciously for as long as it takes to replace old, negative thoughts with a productive, kinder mindset. I know it may feel like a lot of effort, but thoughts control actions. When you control what you think, you can take back control of how you act. The old feelings of frustration will quickly turn into motivation, and your success will be even more rewarding in the end when you put in the work.

DIGGING INTO EMOTIONAL EATING

Rewarding ourselves with food and using it as compensation for challenging events are perhaps the most human of all eating behaviors. Both positive and negative emotions can cause us to crave sugary, greasy food, simply because it feels like a safe and comforting response to stress. And these responses are enforced everywhere we look. How often do you see a woman

make the switch with reframing

Old mindset	New mindset
I must work out twice as long because I ate a chocolate bar.	I enjoyed the chocolate and will use the extra energy for my next workout.
I've now gained a pound because I ate the chocolate bar.	It's normal for my weight to fluctuate based on many things, such as time of day, my water intake, changes in fiber, salt retention, physical activity, and hormones. Gaining a pound doesn't define my journey. My weight doesn't determine my self-worth. The chocolate bar I ate had 250 calories. To realistically gain one pound, I would have to eat fourteen bars.
I have so many other things to prioritize, I can't afford to make time for myself.	My health is nonnegotiable. There's never going to be a more "perfect time" to prioritize my health than today. If I don't do this for myself, no one else will. Taking care of myself will help me become better in other areas of life.
I don't have the time to cook healthy meals during the week.	I will prepare for busy weekdays by making food in larger batches over the weekend. I'm making fueling my body a priority despite my hectic schedule.
I'll gain weight if I don't work out today.	Missing one workout doesn't affect my journey. I'll enjoy taking a rest day and get back to my exercise regimen tomorrow. Taking rest days is just as important as working out.

on a sitcom grabbing a huge glass of wine to deal with the stress going on in her life? Now, I'm not saying the occasional drink is a problem, but it shouldn't be a go-to solution to stress. Removing food or alcohol as a de-stressor is key to dismantling this habit.

Next time you feel like resorting to a bag of chips or a glass of wine as a reward or for comfort, try these instead:

- meet up with a friend
- take a bubble bath
- connect with your *Sculpt* squad
- complete a workout in the app
- try a five-minute meditation (page 99)
- step out for a walk outdoors

INDULGING ON AUTOPILOT

There may be times when you don't feel hungry or even crave food, but you're so used to eating something at a certain time that you indulge simply because it's a habit. Say you sit down to watch your favorite show every Tuesday at 8 p.m. and bring along a bag of chips to snack on. You do it automatically, and often without considering whether you actually *want* chips. Planning out your meals for the day ahead of time and keeping structured mealtimes is a huge help to eliminate habitual snacking. With *Sculpt*, your meals and snacks are scheduled into your Meal Builder in chapter 6.

SAYING GOODBYE TO LATE-NIGHT SNACKING

Many people have a hard time with nighttime snacking as one of their biggest obstacles. Picture this: You start the day strong with a healthy breakfast, a satisfying lunch, and delicious snacks to keep you full in between meals. You get your daily movement in. You've checked all the boxes of a productive day. You're feeling great, as you should!

But as soon as you've had the last meal of the day, all your good intentions go out the window. Why is that? Because at night, many of us indulge as a way to

separating real hunger from emotional hunger

Emotional hunger	Real hunger
I crave specific foods.	Any food that can fill me up will do.
My cravings can't wait.	My cravings can wait.
The hunger appears suddenly.	The hunger develops gradually.
I don't feel full after eating.	I feel full by the time I finish my meal.
I get feelings of guilt or shame after eating.	I feel satisfied after eating.
I'm bored and need a distraction.	My body is giving me physical signals of hunger (e.g., stomach growling).

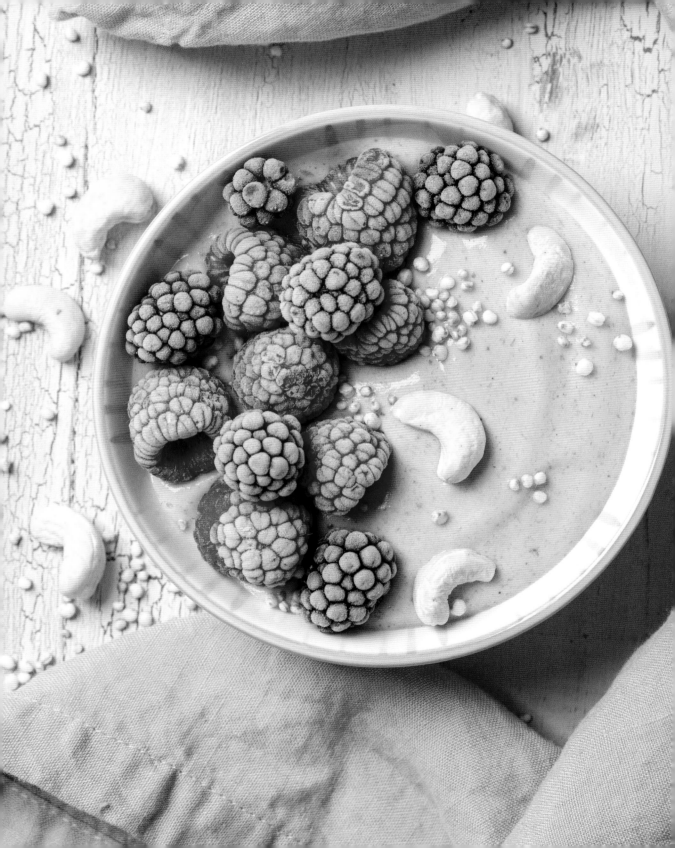

be your own cheerleader

The only person you should compare yourself to is who you were yesterday. You must become your own cheerleader, celebrating every bit of progress that gets you an inch closer to your goals every day. So, rather than focusing on someone else's workout, meal, or life, let's celebrate and enjoy our own journeys!

unwind. While we don't gain more weight from food that's consumed at night—that's a myth—eliminating extra snacking can reduce the total calories you consume in the day. Plus, late-night snacking is the least likely kind of eating to be about hunger. Rather, it is often about boredom—hitting the fridge to binge mindlessly on anything that brings us comfort.

If you struggle with nighttime snacking, try these tips:

CLEAR OUT THE PANTRY! The most effective way to prevent nighttime snacking is by removing packaged foods like candy and potato chips, so you can't resort to eating them out of habit, or boredom. If most of the foods in your home are part of your Meal Builder and food swap tables, then you're already halfway there!

LIST NON-FOOD RELATED STRESS RELIEVERS, like pampering yourself with a bubble bath or doing a skincare night at home. When you get the urge to grab extra snacks, choose one thing from the list instead.

WRITE DOWN WHAT YOU EAT. Accountability plays an important role in weight loss, and studies have shown that keeping a food diary can help you reduce snacking. Although food logging isn't required on the *Sculpt* program, writing down your meals can assist with getting rid of nightly cravings. It can also help you identify other unhelpful patterns that you could benefit from changing.

MAKE SURE YOU'RE DRINKING ENOUGH WATER! Because thirst can sometimes mask itself as hunger, make a habit out of drinking plenty of water with your meals and throughout the day.

the plan after the plan

In the overwhelming majority of cases, the hardest part of weight loss is not actually losing the weight. It's preventing the rebound effect. While there are several factors behind this, including many of the habits we've talked about in this chapter, most diets simply don't come with instructions on what to do after losing weight.

For true, sustainable change, your post-weight-loss plan should be as complete as the period of weight loss itself. That is why the third phase of the *Sculpt* program is dedicated to ensuring your success in the long run by giving you the guidelines to shift your metabolism out of the weight loss mode to a comfortable maintenance level, sticking to the positive habits you've built and avoiding weight regain.

I've introduced you to a lot of new information in this chapter, and different ways of thinking that I hope you'll put into practice. Changing long-ingrained habits and adjusting your mindset can be challenging at first, so refer to this chapter as much as you need to. Revisit the activities and techniques regularly. As you move forward on your journey with *Sculpt,* you'll be forming more and more new lifestyle habits along the way. Remember to make time for some self-care as you put these habits into place—more on that in chapter 9. You're worth it!

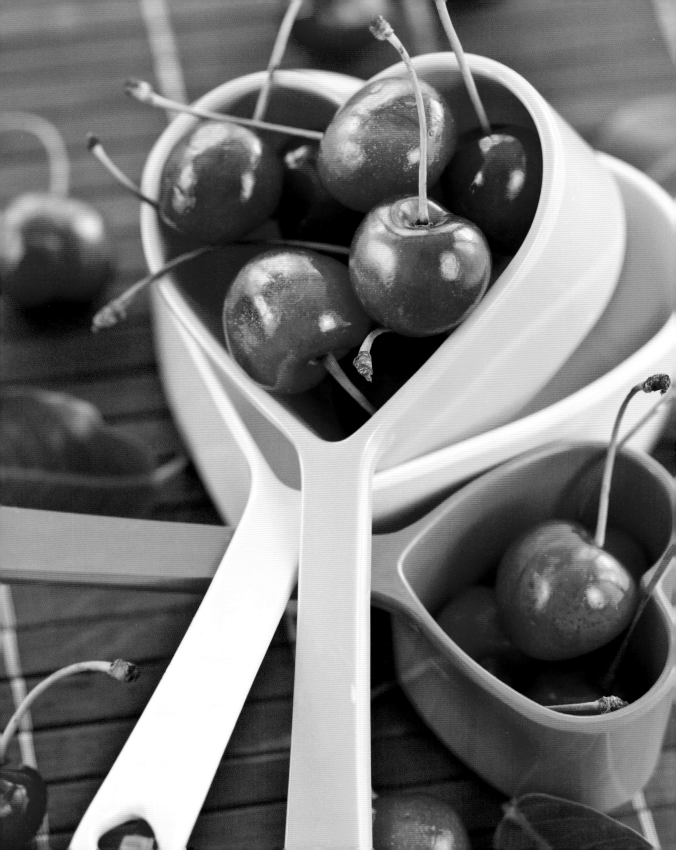

CHAPTER 4

going for the gold

THERE'S SOMETHING THAT YOU AND I have in common. When we led a life of unhealthy, counterproductive habits—past tense, because that's not our reality anymore—a day came when we realized we wanted something better for ourselves. Maybe you're like me and your body was telling you *enough* by forcing you to listen. Or maybe something else sparked a need for change within you. Regardless, there's an area of your life that you want to improve through losing weight, whether it's how you look, your health, or how you feel when you wake up every day. Whatever your reason, we're in this together now!

In this chapter, we will talk about:

- finding the purpose behind your journey
- defining your specific weight loss goals
- learning how to evaluate those goals
- setting SMARTer goals
- tracking your progress accurately
- reevaluating the role of the scale
- creating your list of nonnegotiables

Making a permanent lifestyle change is a positive process, but it's also a long-term commitment. Creating lasting change requires accountability, discipline, and a consistent mindset. Motivation won't always be present. There will be days when you jump out of bed full of energy, and on other days you might not feel like doing anything. To work around the not-so-great days and bounce back stronger, we need a good backup plan.

setting goals for success

Many people fear goal setting because it creates an objective marker for what could be "failure." The problem with that mindset is that it will hold us back from achieving *anything* at all! Setting goals is like drawing a road map for any journey in life. It gives you a sense of direction and drive. And in weight loss, the end goal shouldn't be the number on the scale but what you want to achieve as the result of losing the weight.

Some examples of a specific end goal include:
I want to feel happy with my body.
I want to run my first marathon.
I want to feel confident in my skin.
I want to gain back control of my health.

What do you visualize achieving as the result of your journey? What does success look like for you? Write each of your specific end goals. These will keep you going when the times get tough! And once you understand your larger goals, it will be easier to break them into smaller, more achievable pieces.

Now, let's dig even deeper. Why do you want to achieve these goals? Why does it matter to you? How will they enhance your life? Why is this journey important to you? To stick to the process wholeheartedly, you need a meaningful reason for wanting to tick off the goals on your list. The strength of your reasons behind those goals will determine how consistent you become in your pursuit. Without a clear purpose, you'll likely feel lost and unmotivated sooner than later.

But not every reason is productive. If your goal comes from a place of self-loathing or need for acceptance from others, it will never truly serve you. Take this moment to reflect on your goals and the reasons why you want to achieve them. Be honest and kind to yourself. Focus on moving away from reasons that come from a negative place, and then replace them with kind and empowering ones. Make sure your reasons will support your growth both in the moment and in the future.

Let's revisit your goals. By now, they may look like these:

I WANT TO FEEL CONFIDENT in my skin to enjoy wearing a swimsuit.

I WANT TO BE FIT so I can run around with my kids.

I WANT TO GAIN BACK MY HEALTH to set an example for my family.

Psychologists have spent a lot of time studying the art of goal setting. In my experience, nothing beats the SMART method. SMART stands for specific, measurable, attainable, relevant, and timely. This approach helps ensure your objectives are clearly defined and attainable within a reasonable timeframe.

To turn your goal into a SMART goal, let's make sure it checks each one of these boxes.

SPECIFIC GOALS FOCUS on one milestone you want to reach. Refine your goal to get at what you really want to accomplish and what steps need to be taken to get there. Avoid setting goals that are too broad.

MEASURABLE BENCHMARKS make it easier to track your progress and know when you've reached the finish line.

ATTAINABILITY IS KEY. Your objectives can be ambitious, but they should also be realistic. Ask yourself if this goal is something you can reasonably accomplish.

RELEVANCY: Look at your list of reasons behind why you want to lose weight. Think about the big picture. Why are you setting this goal? Does it fit your plan?

YOU NEED TO SET A TIMEFRAME to measure your progress and success. It's also easier to commit to a goal if you're doing it for a set amount of time. When will you start working toward this goal? When do you want to reach it?

Revisit your goals one more time. If necessary, rewrite them to meet the SMART standards.

FROM SHORT-TERM TO LONG-TERM GOALS

Short-term goals are things you plan to accomplish within a month or two. They may be part of a long-term goal, like losing 5 pounds (2½ kg) in the next month in pursuit of losing 60 pounds (30 kg) in the next year. Short-term goals are smaller and more approachable. They're the goals you should feel relatively confident about achieving.

Long-term goals are things we want to achieve in about a year or more—they are the big, daunting, ambitious goals. It's important to go back and evaluate your short-term goals after the timeframes you've set for them. Sometimes, your short-term goals can help you define what you want from your long-term goals.

Evaluating your goals is a positive thing. If you can tell that you're not reaching your goal, it means that

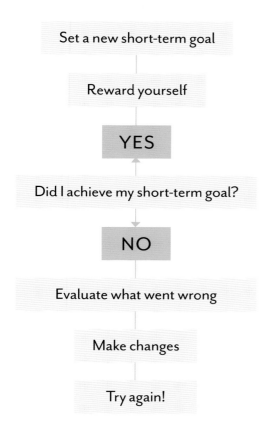

Set a new short-term goal

Reward yourself

YES

Did I achieve my short-term goal?

NO

Evaluate what went wrong

Make changes

Try again!

it's measurable, which allows you to adjust and change your approach. Then you can give it another try!

It's important to remember that when you set your mind to achieving new goals, you're guaranteed to encounter obstacles, feelings of frustration, disruptions, and even failure along the way. This is especially true with big lifestyle changes. It's important, from time to time, to remind yourself about the purpose behind your goals and to not let the setbacks dictate your actions. These are exactly the moments when revisiting your reasons can help you push through challenges.

TRACKING YOUR PROGRESS

Our work together carries on throughout the entire program—and beyond. We start by developing beneficial habits that will help you stay consistent. Here are the most effective ways to self-monitor your progress.

Because of weight plateaus, water retention, menstrual cycles, and natural daily fluctuations that occur in the body, relying too much on a single metric to define progress can be deceiving. And as much as we'd like for the progress to be linear, it often looks more like this:

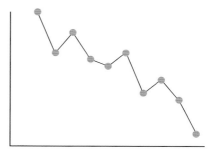

And that's totally normal! In fact, it's part of what will shape your journey. To give you the most accurate snapshot of your progress, *Sculpt* relies on several methods of tracking. You might respond more positively to some than to others, but I encourage you to give them all a chance.

set the stage

There is power in putting your thoughts on paper! It may sound scary to write down your goals, but you are significantly more likely to achieve them by simply writing them down regularly. No one else has to see them, but writing, reading through, and updating your goals can give you an extra boost on days when you're not feeling as motivated.

#1: Take Your Measurements

Did you know that taking your body measurements is one of the most precise methods of tracking? You could weigh the same at two different points in time, but a scale won't reveal changes in your body composition, such as fat loss. Because muscle is denser than fat tissue, measuring tape will show actual inches lost, which is much more exciting than the scale anyway!

After taking your initial measurements with a soft tape, repeat them every two weeks wearing the same or similar clothes. I recommend taking your measurements in underwear or naked for best accuracy.

#2: Weigh Yourself

Over the years, studies have consistently shown that people who weigh themselves regularly tend to be more successful in losing weight in the long term. In this program, we never assess your progress exclusively on the number on the scale; we use it as one of many tools, as well as to determine your water intake needs, group, and maintenance level. After all, the number on the scale is only one indicator of results.

It's normal for your weight to fluctuate throughout the day. This depends on a variety of factors, like how hydrated you are, how much you've eaten and how much sodium that food contained, when you last used the bathroom, and if you recently had an intense workout.

Say you were to weigh yourself in the morning, and again in the afternoon. By then, the number on the scale could have increased by several pounds. Rather than real weight gain, this is part of the body's natural weight fluctuation, and it makes relying solely on the number on the scale inaccurate.

I recommend weighing yourself once a week. If you're used to doing it more often and prefer to continue that way, try limiting it to two or three days distributed across the week (such as Monday, Wednesday, and Friday). Then, calculate your average weekly weight by adding up the recorded weights from each

how to take your measurements

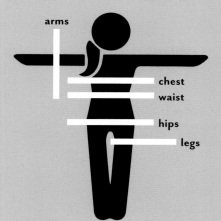

Arms: measure around the widest part of your upper arm

Chest: measure around the widest area of your chest

Waist: measure around your belly button

Hips: measure around the widest area of your butt

Legs: measure around the midpoint of your thigh

Pay attention to where you're measuring each time. You can use any marks on your body as reference points to stay consistent. Make a note and take your measurements from the same spot next time.

day and dividing that number by the number of days you weighed yourself. If you weighed yourself on three days and the scale showed 223, 221, and 220 pounds, add those numbers together (664) and divide the total by three (664/3). Your average weight for the week then becomes 221.3 pounds.

The golden rule is to weigh yourself right after waking up and after you've used the bathroom, before eating or drinking anything. Wear as little clothing as possible—preferably naked or in underwear. To maximize accuracy, place your scale on the same hard, even surface each time you weigh yourself, with your weight distributed evenly on both feet.

No matter how hard you've worked, your weight can sometimes plateau temporarily. As frustrating as it can feel, this is one of the main reasons I don't recommend basing your success only off the scale or weighing yourself daily. If you've experienced scale-dependency or struggled with obsessing over weight in the past, it may be a good idea to put the scale away for now and focus on the other methods of tracking your progress.

#3: Take Progress Photos

Taking before and after photos is the best way to witness progress with your own eyes! My go-to method for taking progress pictures is to record a full-body video in front of a well-lit, plain background holding a natural front, side, and back pose. When you play the video back, you'll be able to take screenshots on your phone. You can also have your partner or friend take pictures of you. Keep your camera angles the same each time and wear similar clothes for an easy progress check!

#4: Start a Bullet Journal

Even if you find that the number on the scale hasn't changed when you weigh yourself, you're still making progress each day. It will all add up! Journaling is a

app check-ins

Through the app (accessible by entering thesculptplan.com/book), you can complete a check-in and collect redeemable points every two weeks! While this is optional, it's a great way to stay on track with your progress. As part of your check-in, you'll weigh yourself, log your measurements, and submit progress photos (also optional).

weight loss or fat loss?

For the sake of clarity, you'll see me refer to *weight loss* throughout this book because that's the term that is commonly used for this journey. But if we want to get technical, is the reduction in body weight actually what we're trying to achieve? For most people who say they want to lose weight, the actual goal is lowering their body fat percentage and achieving an improvement in their body composition. While this does often show as weight loss on the scale, it's also apparent in the way your body looks on the outside. As you reduce your fat mass, your clothes will fit visibly looser.

create your own bullet journal

Think of a bullet journal as a list of nonnegotiable daily goals for the week ahead. It could include moving your body for at least thirty minutes, sticking to regular mealtimes every three to four hours, taking five minutes to meditate, or getting seven to nine hours of sleep. Tick off each day that you complete to keep yourself on track and accountable. When you take your goals day by day, a little becomes a lot!

- improving medical results
- feeling more confident
- stressing less about uncomfortable situations
- developing a positive relationship with food
- eating mindfully
- making healthier choices
- feeling good about life
- discovering new foods
- receiving compliments
- motivating others to live healthier

#6 Keep a Food Log (optional)

As long as you're assembling your meals according to the Meal Builder and sticking to it, logging your foods isn't a must in this program. However, some find it useful to begin with healthy eating habits by keeping a food diary. Although it's a little time-consuming, it's a proven technique; consistent meal logging has been shown to increase the rate of success in weight loss. While this is an optional step, writing down your daily food and drink intake can help you get a better grasp of your true habits and portion sizes as you're getting familiar with them.

powerful place to record your daily wins and progress, and it will give you a full-scale look at your journey. With a bullet journal, you can keep track of your goals, eating and meal planning, movement, sleep, water intake, and self-care. Use the next page to start your own bullet journal!

#5: Celebrate Non-Scale Wins

Remember to celebrate all of those accomplishments that can't be measured in numbers! We often forget about our non-scale wins, even though they're such a big part of the journey. These victories may seem small, but they are where you really see the impact of your consistent efforts and new habits.

Non-scale wins can include:

- having more energy
- sleeping better
- feeling more comfortable in your clothes
- completing a full workout without getting tired
- exercising with more intensity
- using heavier weights

when not to track

To avoid feelings of frustration, I don't recommend taking your measurements, progress photos or weighing yourself on the days leading up to and during your period. Bloating, water retention, and hormonal changes can often cause a temporary weight gain of 3 to 5 pounds (1 to 3 kg). On these days, stick to other methods and celebrate your non-scale wins!

bullet journal and progress tracker

S	M	T	W	T	F	S	Weekly goals and nonnegotiables
○	○	○	○	○	○	○	
○	○	○	○	○	○	○	
○	○	○	○	○	○	○	
○	○	○	○	○	○	○	
○	○	○	○	○	○	○	
○	○	○	○	○	○	○	
○	○	○	○	○	○	○	
○	○	○	○	○	○	○	
○	○	○	○	○	○	○	
○	○	○	○	○	○	○	
○	○	○	○	○	○	○	
○	○	○	○	○	○	○	
○	○	○	○	○	○	○	
○	○	○	○	○	○	○	
○	○	○	○	○	○	○	
○	○	○	○	○	○	○	
○	○	○	○	○	○	○	
○	○	○	○	○	○	○	
○	○	○	○	○	○	○	
○	○	○	○	○	○	○	

Progress tracker

Weight: Arms:

Chest: Waist:

Hips: Legs:

set

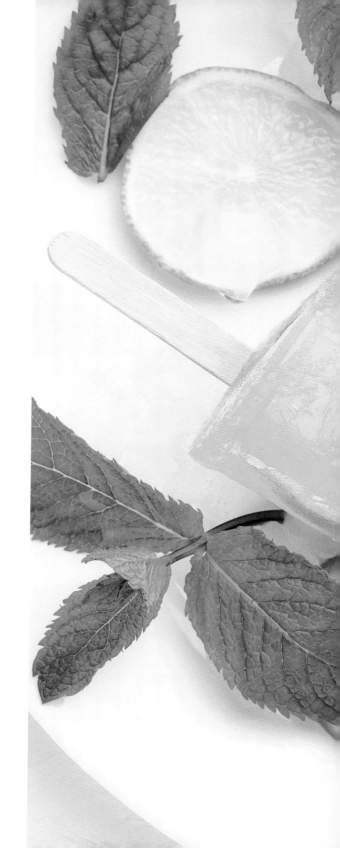

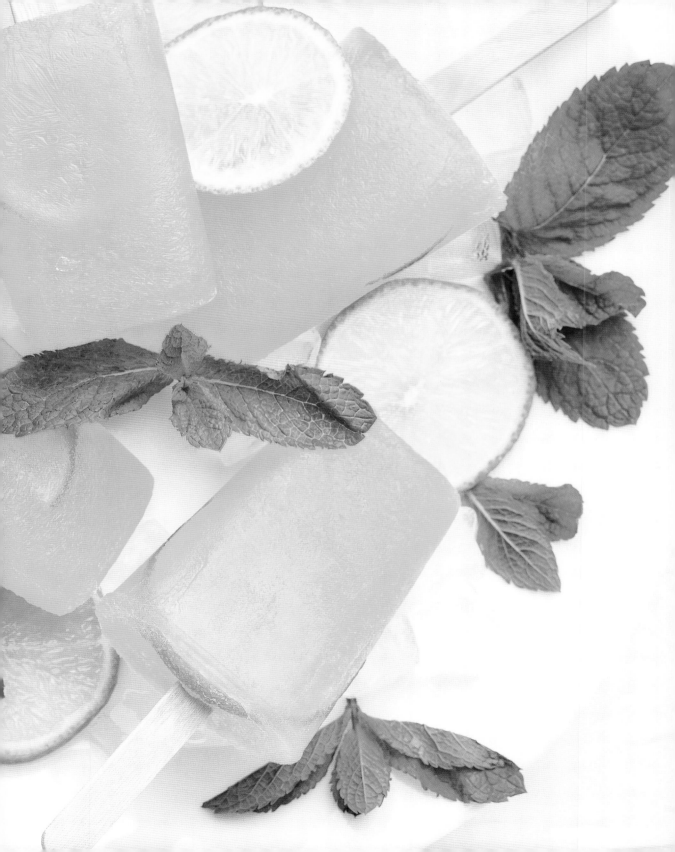

eating to lose weight

DID YOU KNOW THAT THE MAJORITY of Americans are malnourished? You can be malnourished even if you eat plenty of food—it just means that you're not getting enough *nutritious* food. We are constantly surrounded by food choices, and it's no wonder we often feel like we're doing it all wrong with so much contradictory information about what we should and shouldn't eat. In this chapter, I share everything you need to know about nutrition, so you can keep making smart food choices for the rest of your life!

After this chapter, you'll be able to:

- begin repairing a sluggish metabolism
- identify foods that will benefit your journey
- make smarter choices at the grocery store
- understand your Meal Builder options and why they work

What we eat is undoubtedly the most crucial component of any weight loss program. But good nutrition affects much more than weight; it can give us a sharp mind, improved mood, increased energy levels, and glowing skin, just for starters!

healing your metabolism

Your metabolism is the mechanism in charge of breaking down the calories you eat and drink into energy. Your total daily energy expenditure measures how many calories the body burns in a day. That includes both the calories you burn at rest, known as the basal metabolic rate, and the calories you burn through exercise and general moving about. The body burns calories at rest by maintaining cellular function and executing vital tasks, such as keeping the heart beating and regulating body temperature.

Everyone has a different basal metabolic rate, which depends mainly on gender, height, weight, and age. It accounts for about 60 to 80 percent of your total energy expenditure on any given day. Every time you eat, you give your metabolism a nudge. This is because of a process called the thermic effect of food, which accounts for about 10 percent of your overall energy expenditure. It's the energy the body uses for the digestion, absorption, and distribution of nutrients. So, while it may sound counterintuitive, we actually burn calories when we consume food.

Chances are that you have felt the frustration of not being able to lose weight, no matter how hard you try. What worked for you in the past isn't giving you results.

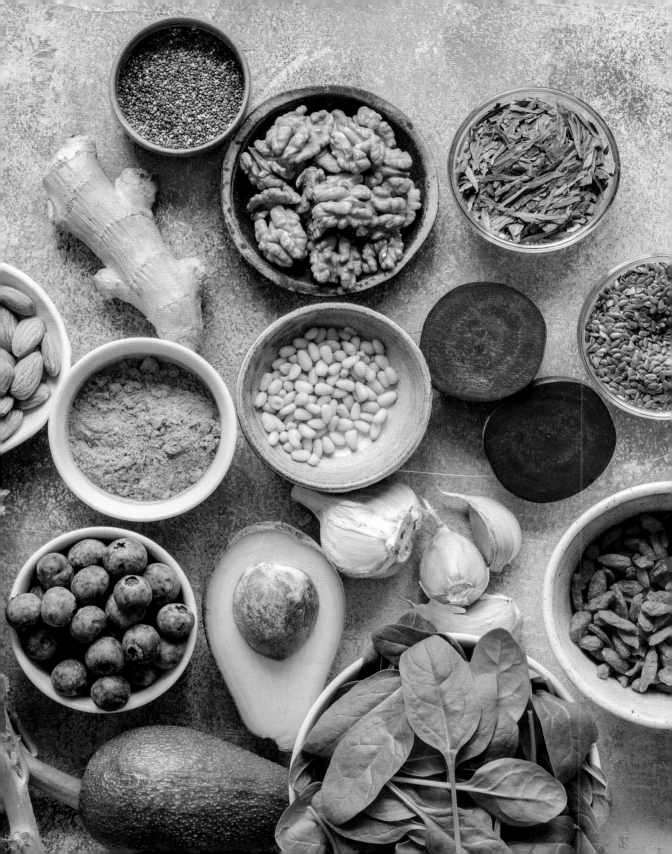

If you've gone through many restrictive diets, your metabolism may have become effectively nonresponsive to quick weight loss efforts. This is called metabolic adaptation, and it happens when you feed your body very little food during restrictive diets, causing your metabolic rate to slow.

The most common factors behind a slowed-down metabolism are:

- extreme calorie restriction for extended periods of time
- yo-yo dieting
- irregular mealtimes
- hormonal changes
- lack of sleep
- drinking too little water
- chronic stress
- certain medications

We're going to dive deeper into metabolic adaptation in chapter 10. For now, the good news is that we have ways of fixing a sluggish metabolism. These include:

- eating more (yes, you read that right!)
- incorporating more protein and fiber in your meals
- getting a solid seven to nine hours of rest per night
- varying your workouts and their intensity
- drinking plenty of water throughout the day
- finding new ways to control stress (put the tips in chapter 9 to test!)

BREAKING DOWN CALORIES

Think of calories as your body's fuel. One pound of body fat contains approximately 3,500 calories. Food can be divided into three macronutrient groups: proteins, carbohydrates, and fats. A gram of protein or carbohydrate contains 4 calories, whereas a gram of fat contains 9 calories. You won't be required to do any calorie counting or macronutrient distribution in this program, but understanding the role of calories and macros sets you up for success when making choices on your own based on nutrition labels.

meet macronutrients

Many diets seek to eliminate a specific macronutrient, but each food group has an equally significant role in maintaining a healthy, sustainable way of eating. Your macronutrients are balanced for you in the next chapter, so you can focus on feeling better inside and out while revving your metabolism!

protein

Protein has a special role in weight loss. First, increasing your daily intake of protein boosts your metabolism and helps you burn more calories throughout the day. Plus, increasing protein helps you feel full longer, resulting in fewer cravings and staving off the insulin spikes that often drive us to snack more in between meals. Of all macronutrients, protein has been shown to cause the largest rise in the thermic effect of food. Protein requires more energy to digest than carbohydrates, meaning that your body will work harder and burn extra calories to break it into energy.

Some protein sources you'll find in your Meal Builder include:

- chicken
- turkey
- fish
- shrimp
- beef
- pork
- eggs

- yogurt
- milk
- tofu
- tempeh
- seitan
- beans
- protein powder

carbohydrates

Many diet trends since the 1990s have shared the same message: Say no to carbs. I'm happy to tell you that isn't the case here! There is absolutely no reason you should fear eating carbs. The idea that you'd need to cut an entire food group from your diet to magically melt away pounds is a total myth—plus, avoiding carbs forever is simply not sustainable for most people.

Did you know that carbohydrates are your body's most important source of fuel? Complex mechanisms like the nervous system, the brain, muscles, and red blood cells all need carbohydrates to function properly. Carbs also play a key role in fat-burning processes.

We often think of grains like pasta, rice, and bread when talking about carbs, but fruit and vegetables are natural sources of carbohydrate, too. We get all our fiber from carbohydrates; fiber keeps us feeling full and going to the bathroom regularly. And of course, carbs are delicious, which is another good reason to keep them around!

Now, that's not to say that all carbohydrates are created equal, or that eating supersized portions that are high in added sugars or empty calories won't affect your weight loss. We can enjoy all food groups in smart amounts that help us get closer to our goals. The carbohydrate group can be divided into simple and complex. Simple carbohydrates are sugars and processed grains like white bread, crackers, chips, white pasta, white rice, sweet desserts, and candy, which *can* sabotage your progress if simple carbs are the only type of carbs you consume. They digest quickly and have a high glycemic index (GI) score, causing spikes in your blood sugar levels followed by a sudden drop in energy. This cycle of blood sugar spikes can lead to overeating and cravings. Although simple carbs like white rice and spaghetti won't keep you full for as long as whole grains, and provide fewer nutrients, it's perfectly fine to incorporate them a few times a week if you enjoy having them.

Complex carbohydrates, or smart carbs as they're often called, are carbohydrates that the body digests slowly. They are nutrient-rich and full of fiber. These carbohydrates include brown rice, whole wheat bread, oats, starchy vegetables, legumes like beans and lentils, nuts, and seeds. They fill us up, but unlike simple carbs, they won't spike your insulin levels, instead providing a steady stream of fuel to power through the day. That's why complex carbs are the preferred everyday source of starch in your food swap tables, starting on page 64.

fiber-packed options

Try incorporating some of these foods into your meals for a boost of extra fiber:

- artichokes
- raspberries
- black beans
- blackberries
- chickpeas
- chia seeds
- broccoli
- avocados
- apples
- oatmeal
- almonds
- flaxseed

introducing the glycemic index

You may have heard about the glycemic index, a system that measures how much a certain food or drink boosts blood sugar. Carbohydrates ranked with a high score cause your blood sugar to spike quickly;

those with a lower score have a much slower and less significant effect. It's important to note that this categorization doesn't necessarily label foods as "bad," or "prohibited." In fact, you will see some of the higher-scoring foods as options in your food swaps.

LOW GI FOODS

apples	brown rice
berries	whole-grain pasta
peaches	muesli
oranges	mushrooms
tomatoes	carrots
lemons	green peas
broccoli	black beans
cauliflower	lentils
cucumbers	chickpeas
lettuce	cashews
kale	peanuts
onions	yogurt
boiled sweet potatoes	corn

MEDIUM GI FOODS

pineapples	basmati rice
kiwi fruit	crispbreads
white rice	unsweetened cereal
beetroot	whole wheat bread
pita bread	couscous

HIGH GI FOODS

watermelon	corn flakes
baked potatoes	pretzels
rice cakes	jellybeans
white bread	donuts

instead of this, try that!

White rice	Brown rice, wild rice, cauliflower rice
White pasta	Whole wheat pasta, brown rice pasta, wild rice pasta
White bread	Whole-grain bread, sprouted grain bread
Instant oats	Old-fashioned rolled oats
Potato chips with dip	Veggie sticks with dip
All-purpose flour	Almond flour, coconut flour, ground oats
Dried fruit	Fresh fruit
Sugary cereals	Oatmeal, unsweetened cereal, corn flakes
Pizza crust	Pita bread, tortilla wrap, cauliflower crust
Breadcrumbs	Ground oats

focus on fiber

Like protein, fiber is your ticket to feeling full and satisfied after a meal. We want to aim for at least 25 grams of fiber per day. Besides promoting regularity, getting enough fiber helps keep your blood sugar steady so you can stay focused and productive all day.

Fiber is naturally found in the cell walls of plants, so by choosing more plant-based options, you'll automatically increase your fiber intake. Fruit, vegetables, legumes, and whole grains have the highest fiber content—eating more of them will show on the inside and out!

fat

Before carbohydrates became the bad guys, fats were labeled as the enemy to avoid at all costs. It's funny to think about now because we know that eating the right fats in the right amounts is crucial to looking and feeling amazing. That's right, we need fat to burn fat!

Your brain demands essential fatty acids omega-3 and omega-6 from your diet to function properly—in fact, did you know that about 60 percent of your brain is made of fat? Fats also play a key role in facilitating the absorption of vitamins A, D, E, and K. Not to mention, an appropriate amount of healthy fats will have your skin glowing, your hair and nails shiny and strong, and your mood and energy levels up. Out of all the macronutrients, fats take the longest for the body to digest—and they make food taste so much better!

When selecting between different fats, we will opt for unsaturated fat whenever possible. These healthy fats include:

- avocados
- fatty fish
- extra-virgin olive oil
- olives
- egg yolks
- nuts
- nut butters
- seeds

Saturated fat, found in foods such as butter, coconut oil, whole milk dairy, and red meat, is a type of dietary fat that should be consumed in moderation, as it can make your cholesterol levels higher and increase the risk of heart disease. However, it can be enjoyed here and there. The American Heart Association recommends limiting saturated fat intake to 5 to 6 percent of total calories per day. For this reason, you'll notice that in your swap tables, foods that are high in saturated fat are listed separately, and low-fat and fat-free versions of dairy products are preferred over full-fat options.

There is one type of fat that should *always* be skipped. Trans fats, which are banned by the U.S. Food and Drug Administration (FDA), are linked to many negative health effects such as heart disease, increased cholesterol levels, and increased inflammation. They raise your "bad" cholesterol and lower your "good" cholesterol. Watch out for trans fats in fried and fast foods, chips, and ready-made frozen meals.

don't forget micronutrients

In addition to macronutrients, we get micronutrients—better known as vitamins and minerals—from food. Vitamins and minerals don't contain any calories, and your body needs them in much smaller quantities. All micronutrients play an essential role in vital functions of the body, as well as your overall health. Therefore, it's very important that you get the recommended values from food and by boosting your diet with supplements, if needed. While vitamins and minerals alone won't produce weight loss, there are certain micronutrients, such as magnesium and vitamins B and D, that have been linked to functions that can aid it.

LOW-FAT OR FAT-FREE ALTERNATIVES

Be mindful when reading the nutrition labels of a lighter version of a product. The FDA regulates label claims as follows:

- **FAT-FREE** means 0.5 grams of fat or less per serving
- **LOW-FAT** means 3 grams of fat or less per serving

instead of this, try that!

Bacon	Turkey bacon
Ice cream	Homemade sorbet, frozen yogurt, nice cream
Full-fat dairy	Plant-based nut milks, low-fat and fat-free dairy
French fries	Crispy Air-Fryer Fries (page 184), sweet potato wedges
Beef Bolognese	Turkey Bolognese, tofu Bolognese

can diet sodas make you gain weight?

Directly, no. Diet sodas are usually free of calories, or low-calorie alternatives to sugary beverages, but that doesn't necessarily mean there's no link to weight. That said, some studies suggest that artificial sweeteners may make you hungrier by increasing your appetite, which could lead to overeating and weight gain. Because diet sodas carry no nutritional value, it's smart to consider limiting them.

- **REDUCED FAT** must have at least 25 percent less fat than the regular product

- **LIGHT** must have 1/3 fewer calories, or at least 50 percent less fat than the regular product

To make up for the lower fat content, some items include additives to make up for the flavor and texture lost in the fat-removing process; this can sneakily add to their calorie content.

First, make sure that the item is actually lower in calories than the regular product. You'd be surprised—that's not always the case! Then, check if the marked serving sizes are the same for both options. A label could show a lower calorie content, but for a different serving size! Certain items, like most low-fat and fat-free dairy products, are good options given

the reduced saturated fat content compared to their whole-fat dairy counterparts.

the role of hydration

Drinking enough water may not be the most inspiring part of a healthy lifestyle, and because of that it's one that is often forgotten. While drinking water won't produce weight loss on its own, it can help. Fluids play a vital role in important metabolic processes, such as the digestion of food and dissolving water-soluble vitamins, and proper hydration is necessary for your body to function as it's supposed to. Water helps the kidneys flush toxins from your body. Without enough water in your system, the waste can't get out as it should, causing the body to hold onto toxins instead of releasing them.

One of the first signs that you're not drinking enough water is fatigue and irritability. That mid-afternoon energy slump could be simply because you're not getting enough fluids! Thirst can also disguise itself as hunger, and it's easier to give into comfort foods and sugary cravings when you're even slightly dehydrated.

The rule of thumb is to aim for eight glasses of water a day. To figure out exactly what your daily fluid intake should be, take your weight in pounds and divide it by 2. That's the number of ounces you'll want to aim for each day. For example, if you weigh 200 pounds, you'll need to drink 100 ounces (about 3 L). Factors like intense exercise and hot weather will increase the need to replenish fluid loss and hydrate more. When working out, add at least 17 ounces (½ L) of water to your daily hydration goal.

let's talk labels

Whether you're consciously looking at food labels or not, you're surrounded by them every single day. Some claims on food are strictly regulated by the government, whereas others are used only for marketing purposes and can sometimes be misleading. To make well-informed decisions while grocery shopping, it's important to understand the definitions of commonly used product labels and markings.

GMOs: Genetically modified organisms are living organisms that have had their DNA modified in a laboratory in a targeted way. Usually, this has been done by adding genes from another organism. Some foods that commonly use GMOs are corn, soybeans, and canola. Using GMOs in food is problematic because there's a lot that scientists still don't know about how our bodies react to genetically modified food. Some suspect it may lead to allergies, infertility, and even cancer.

Organic: Organic food is grown by farmers or food producers without most conventional pesticides. Does that mean that it's grown without any chemicals? Not

making meals more plant-based

A plant-based diet is heavy on produce and richer in micronutrients, such as vitamins C and E, fiber, folic acid, potassium, and magnesium. It's no wonder that a plant-based diet not only reduces inflammation, but it also lowers the rate of heart disease, diabetes, and cancer. Even if you're not vegetarian or vegan, try incorporating more plant-based options throughout the week by looking for swap items marked with V+, or set a goal of eating plant-based one day out of the week!

necessarily. In fact, almost no food is 100 percent free of pesticides. Organic food is produced without fertilizer using synthetic ingredients, sewage sludge, bioengineering, or ionizing radiation. But there are natural and synthetic pesticides that can still be used on organic produce under the law. Certain pesticides are linked to many chronic diseases, including fertility problems, hormonal issues, diabetes, asthma, and cancer.

Pasture-raised: A pasture-raised label is commonly found on eggs, dairy, poultry, and beef. It refers to animals that were raised grazing on pasture, or with access to a pasture, instead of being permanently confined indoors. However, they may have been fed supplemental grain as part of their diet.

Grass-fed: Grass-fed labels are common in beef and dairy products, and they refer to animals that were raised on pasture.

Antibiotic-free: No antibiotics were administered to the animal during its lifetime.

Cage-free: Eggs marked as "cage-free" come from cage-free chickens, meaning they have a minimum of 1¼ square foot of space to move. Cage-free doesn't necessarily mean that the chickens can roam around freely.

Free-range: Much like cage-free chickens, free-range chickens ostensibly don't have to live in confinement and can go outside. However, the only real requirement for the "free-range" label is that the facility has a door to 21.8 square feet (2 sq m) of outdoor space—which doesn't automatically mean that chickens actually spend time outside.

Farmed: Farm-raised seafood means fish and shellfish that are raised in controlled waters or factory tanks. More than half of the seafood available in America is farmed.

Wild-caught: Seafood that has been caught from its natural habitat—a lake, river, or the ocean.

No added hormones: This label indicates that the animal was not administered any synthetic hormones. This is not actually that remarkable because adding hormones to any poultry, hog, or bison products is prohibited in the United States at the federal level. However, many companies use the label as a marketing technique.

Humanely raised: This label has quite a vague definition, and it is only certified by third parties rather than by any government agency. It often describes animals that were raised on pasture in an ethical fashion with minimal stress and unlimited access to food and water, without antibiotics or hormones being administered.

what to avoid and why

As you may have guessed from the foods we've looked at in this chapter, the *Sculpt* way of eating opts for

what produce should i buy organic?

When it comes to produce, organic options are often more expensive, and you may not find an organic option for every fruit and vegetable in the produce aisle. I find it useful to keep track of the Dirty Dozen and Clean 15 lists to help me decide when to buy organic, and when it's fine to buy conventional. The Dirty Dozen lists foods that are considered as the most pesticide-heavy produce items available in American grocery stores. Items under the Dirty Dozen list are my nonnegotiables that I'd rather replace with something similar, unless I can find an organic version. The list changes periodically, but it traditionally includes strawberries, apples, spinach, grapes, cherries, pears, peaches, nectarines, and peppers. Similarly, the Clean 15 lists the fruit and vegetables with the lowest concentration of pesticides. These typically include avocados, onions, pineapple, broccoli, mushrooms, and cauliflower.

nutrient-rich whole foods over prepackaged and ultra-processed items. Before I continue, did you know that the term "processed" actually refers to any alteration from the food's natural state, including washing, cutting, canning, or freezing? So, not all processed options are negative, and it's challenging to completely avoid processed foods. If buying pre-chopped, frozen, or canned foods is a convenient option that removes a barrier for you to include more non-starchy veggies on your plate, I'm all for it!

Ultra-processed foods, on the other hand, are pre-packaged foods that are significantly associated with weight gain and overweight. These foods are often heavy on chemicals, which may lead to confusion with the body's internal satiety cues. That's why we limit fried, ultra-processed, and chemical-filled foods that don't contribute to our health in any way. These include foods with high fructose corn syrup like cookies, candy, soda, chips, and frozen dinners. As a good rule of thumb, most items that are prepackaged and sold in a bag or box usually fall under the ultra-processed category.

Like all other things, the use of alcohol is a balancing act. You can enjoy an occasional drink on a night out without it hindering your progress, but I recommend keeping alcohol to a minimum, especially during the Set phase. It's easy to forget about sneaky liquid calories, but they can quickly add up if consumed regularly—at 7 calories per gram, alcohol is casually known as the "fourth macronutrient," containing almost twice as many calories per gram as protein or carbs, and nearly as many calories per gram as fat. As far as sweeteners go, minimize beverages with artificial sweeteners such as aspartame, and choose plant-derived sweeteners like stevia, maple syrup, and honey instead.

Having a healthy relationship with eating starts with knowing how to select foods that benefit your journey and contribute to your goals. It's also about recognizing that an occasional treat won't make or break your progress. This has been an information-packed chapter, but don't worry. While you adhere to your Meal Builder guidelines and swap tables in the next chapter, you won't have to figure out the nutritional value of different foods—it's all done for you!

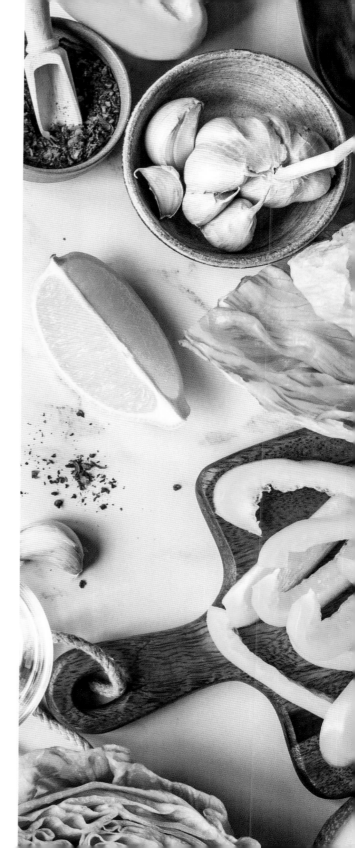

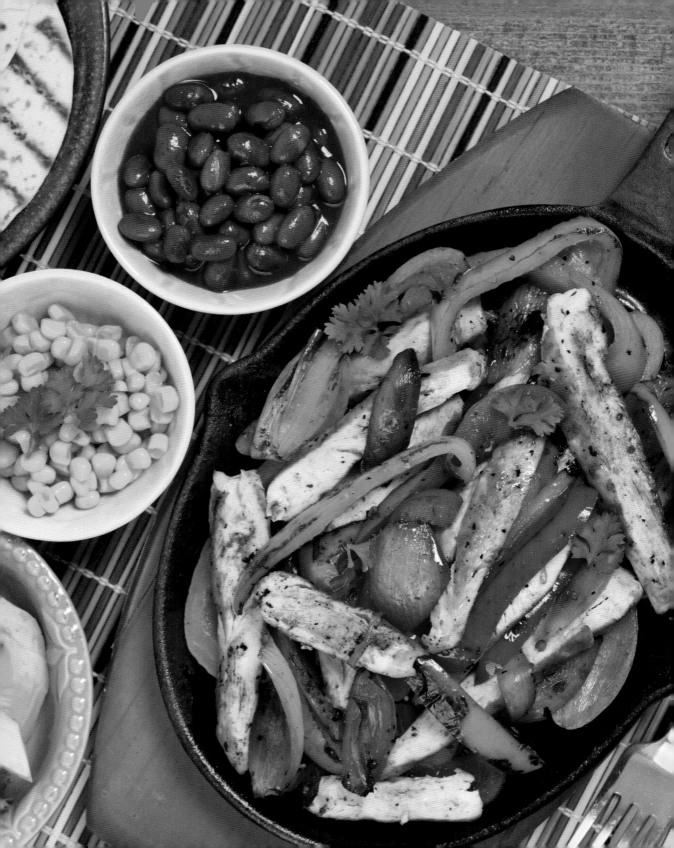

meet the meal builder

THE RIGHT NUTRITION MAKES AN enormous difference for your weight, your health, and how great you feel. This chapter is the heart of the program where you'll apply everything you've learned so far to get closer to the goals you've set, and begin dramatically improving the quality of your life. Even better, you will rediscover the joy of eating and reap the benefits of foods that strengthen your journey. And you'll do it all without counting calories or figuring out what you should eat—so you can focus on what's meaningful, living your life to the fullest!

introducing the meal builder

Unlike most weight loss programs and meal guides, the Meal Builder's balanced portion swap system focuses on guiding you toward positive eating patterns without boxing you in. There are limitless ways to change up your meals, so you never feel bored. It's designed to fit your personal choices because you should have the opportunity to eat the foods you love with zero compromises.

YOUR MEALS AT A GLANCE

Eat Five Meals a Day

No matter what group you belong to, your Meal Builder includes five meals and snacks a day: breakfast, AM snack, lunch, PM snack, and dinner. You get guidelines for portions and options on how to fill your plate with hundreds of alternatives!

No Longer than Three to Four Hours Between Meals

In the *Sculpt* program, your eating schedule is important. To give the body food to burn on a frequent basis and keep blood sugar from plummeting, aim to eat every three to four hours without extra snacking between meals and snacks. If needed, you can switch them around as best fits your schedule.

Eat Your Breakfast by 9 a.m.

Have the first meal of the day before 9 a.m. each day— preferably within thirty minutes of rising. If you wake up after nine o'clock, keep the same schedule starting with breakfast shortly after waking up. A nutritious breakfast refuels your body and sets you up for better eating choices for the rest of the day. Making a routine out of consistent mealtimes helps keep your energy levels up, uninterrupted, all day long. By structuring your meals this way, you're making sure that your blood sugar levels stay steady from morning to night.

Last Meal of the Day by 10 p.m.

If your first meal of the day has taken place early in the morning, you're likely going to eat before 10 p.m. Go by your own schedule and note that you don't have to wait until it's ten o'clock to eat! This is the latest recommended time for your last meal. If your days are irregular or much longer than average, see the frequently asked questions on page 14 for guidance.

find your group

GROUP 1: 1–19 pounds (1–9 kg) to lose

GROUP 2: 20–39 pounds (10–19 kg) to lose

GROUP 3: 40–60 pounds (20–30 kg) to lose

If you need help choosing your group, use the Find My Group table on page 20 for reference. If your goal is to lose more than 60 pounds (30 kg), follow the Meal Builder for Group 3, and choose one add-on to incorporate into your daily meals for every additional 20 pounds (10 kg) or less you want to lose. You'll find the list of add-ons under the Meal Builder for Group 3 (page 61).

You may need to switch between groups as you progress. Here's how that might look:

Example 1: Jennifer wants to lose 60 pounds (30 kg). She follows the Meal Builder for Group 3 until she has lost 21 pounds (11 kg). Then, she switches to Group 2 for the remaining 39 pounds (19 kg). When she's down to losing her last 19 pounds (9 kg), she switches to Group 1 where she stays until she reaches her goal weight.

Example 2: Marissa wants to lose 65 pounds (32 kg). She follows the Meal Builder for Group 3 and enjoys one add-on from the list each day until she has lost 5 pounds (2 kg). From that day on, she continues following the guidelines for Group 3 without additional add-ons. She will continue the program and switch to Group 2 for the remaining 39 pounds (19 kg). When she's down to losing her last 19 pounds (9 kg), she switches to Group 1 where she stays until she reaches her goal weight.

Example 3: Vanessa wants to lose 100 pounds (45 kg). She will follow the Meal Builder for Group 3 and select two add-ons from the list each day, until she has 80 pounds (40 kg) left to lose. From there, she will continue choosing one add-on each day until she has 60 pounds (30 kg) left to lose. Then, she will follow the Group 3 Meal Builder without any add-ons. She will continue the program and switch to Group 2 for the remaining 39 pounds (19 kg). When she's down to losing her last 19 pounds (9 kg), she switches to Group 1, where she stays until she reaches her goal weight.

what's in a portion?

Think of portions as the building blocks of a well-rounded meal. A portion is a pre-calculated amount of an individual food that helps you build balanced meals. Each food on the swap lists is categorized by its nutritional quality. You'll see that foods with high-quality nutrients are on the top of the list in green and recommended for any day, while foods in orange that have a lower nutritional value due to a higher saturated fat content, added sugars, or lower fiber can still be enjoyed in a balanced way.

You'll also notice that often your meals will consist of more than one portion of the same food group. For example, a meal could look like this: 1 portion of starch, 3 portions of protein, and 2 portions of fat. This indicates that you will choose any 1 portion from the starch group, 3 portions from the protein group, and 2 portions from the fat group.

group 1: meal builder

To build your meals, select sample foods for starches, proteins, fats, and fruit based on the number of portions indicated at the bottom of the page. Then, complete your plate with unlimited non-starchy veggies! For a full list of options, choose from swap lists for each food group on pages 64-67.

Starch *1 portion*	1 toast 1 tortilla ½ cup cooked rice 1 small potato	1 small sweet potato ½ cup canned beans ⅓ cup rolled oats ½ cup cooked quinoa	½ cup cooked pasta 1 small pita bread ¼ cup granola 1 cup corn flakes

Protein
1 portion
	1 small egg
	1 ounce cooked chicken breast
	1 ounce cooked lean
	  ground beef
	2 ounces cooked cod
		1 ounce cooked lean
		  turkey breast
		1 ounce cooked salmon
		⅓ cup nonfat greek yogurt
		2 ounces cooked shrimp
			1 ounce cooked lean steak
			1 slice firm tofu
			2 slices turkey bacon
			1 tablespoon protein powder
			2 ounces tuna in water

Fat *1 portion*	1 teaspoon extra-virgin olive oil ¼ small avocado ½ tablespoon peanut butter	1 tablespoon chia seeds 2 tablespoons shredded cheese	2 tablespoons cacao powder 6 almonds ½ tablespoon unsalted butter
Fruit *1 portion*	1 small orange ½ cup mixed berries ½ small banana	1 cup strawberries 1 small peach ½ cup pineapple	1 cup watermelon ½ cup mango ½ cup grapes
Non-starchy vegetables *Unlimited*	tomatoes bell pepper broccoli cauliflower	cucumber green beans lettuce mushrooms	onion spinach carrots collard greens

Breakfast	AM Snack	Lunch	PM Snack	Dinner
1 portion starch 2 portions protein 1 portion fat 1 portion fruit	1 portion starch 1 portion protein 1 portion fat	1½ portions starch 3 portions protein 2 portions fat	2 portions protein 1 portion fruit	1 portion starch 3 portions protein 1 portion fat

+ unlimited non-starchy vegetables

group 2: meal builder

To build your meals, select sample foods for starches, proteins, fats, and fruit based on the number of portions indicated at the bottom of the page. Then, complete your plate with unlimited non-starchy veggies! For a full list of options, choose from swap lists for each food group on pages 64-67.

Starch *1 portion*	1 toast 1 tortilla ½ cup cooked rice 1 small potato	1 small sweet potato ½ cup canned beans ⅓ cup rolled oats ½ cup cooked quinoa	½ cup cooked pasta 1 small pita bread ¼ cup granola 1 cup corn flakes

Protein
1 portion
	1 small egg
	1 ounce cooked chicken breast
	1 ounce cooked
	   lean ground beef
	2 ounces cooked cod
		1 ounce cooked lean
		   turkey breast
		1 ounce cooked salmon
		⅓ cup nonfat greek yogurt
		2 ounces cooked shrimp
			1 ounce cooked lean steak
			1 slice firm tofu
			2 slices turkey bacon
			1 tablespoon protein powder
			2 ounces tuna in water

Fat *1 portion*	1 teaspoon extra-virgin olive oil ¼ small avocado ½ tablespoon peanut butter	1 tablespoon chia seeds 2 tablespoons shredded cheese	2 tablespoons cacao powder ½ tablespoon unsalted butter 6 almonds
Fruit *1 portion*	1 small orange ½ cup mixed berries ½ small banana	1 cup strawberries 1 small peach ½ cup pineapple	1 cup watermelon ½ cup mango ½ cup grapes
Non-starchy vegetables *Unlimited*	tomatoes bell pepper broccoli cauliflower cabbage	cucumber green beans lettuce mushrooms onion	spinach carrots collard greens asparagus scallions

Breakfast	AM Snack	Lunch	PM Snack	Dinner
1 portion starch 3 portions protein 1 portion fat 1 portion fruit	1 portion starch 1 portion protein 1 portion fat	2 portions starch 4 portions protein 2 portions fat	2 portions protein 1 portion fruit	1 portion starch 3 portions protein 2 portions fat

+ unlimited non-starchy vegetables

group 3: meal builder

To build your meals, select sample foods for starches, proteins, fats, and fruit based on the number of portions indicated at the bottom of the page. Then, complete your plate with unlimited non-starchy veggies! For a full list of options, choose from swap lists for each food group on pages 64-67.

Starch *1 portion*	1 toast 1 tortilla	1 small sweet potato ½ cup canned beans	½ cup cooked pasta 1 small pita bread
Protein *1 portion*	1 small egg 1 ounce cooked chicken breast	1 ounce cooked salmon ⅓ cup nonfat greek yogurt	1 ounce cooked lean steak 1 slice firm tofu
Fat *1 portion*	1 teaspoon extra-virgin olive oil ¼ small avocado	2 tablespoons shredded coconut	2 tablespoons cacao powder ½ tablespoon peanut butter
Fruit *1 portion*	1 small orange ½ cup mixed berries	1 cup strawberries 1 small peach	1 cup watermelon ½ cup pineapple
Non-starchy vegetables *Unlimited*	tomatoes bell pepper broccoli	cucumber green beans lettuce	spinach carrots onions

Breakfast	AM Snack	Lunch	PM Snack	Dinner
1 portion starch 3 portions protein 2 portions fat 1 portion fruit	1 portion starch 1 portion protein 1 portion fat	2 portions starch 4 portions protein 2 portions fat	2 portions protein 1 portion fruit	1 portion starch 4 portions protein 3 portions fat

+ unlimited non-starchy vegetables

Select one daily add-on for every additional 20 pounds (10 kg):

Option 1: *1 portion starch*

Option 2: *2 portions protein*

Option 3: *2 portions fat*

Option 4: *1 portion protein + 1 portion fat*

Option 5: *½ portion starch + 1 portion fat*

Option 6: *½ portion starch + 1 portion protein*

Option 7: *2 portions fruit*

Option 8: *1 portion fruit + 1 portion protein*

Option 9: *1 portion fruit + 1 potion fat*

Option 10: *1 portion fruit + ½ portion starch*

dietary restrictions

Look for these icons in the swap tables and recipes to choose the options that best fit your eating style.

S **Standard**
A variety of foods from every food group, and the best fit if you don't have any special food preferences or restrictions.

DF **Dairy-free**
Foods that contain no animal milk and no products made using animal milk. With packaged goods, be sure to double-check the food label of your selected brand to ensure that the product is truly dairy-free.

GF **Gluten-free**
Foods that traditionally contain no wheat, barley, or rye. With packaged goods, be sure to double-check the food label of your selected brand to ensure that the product is truly gluten-free.

V **Vegetarian**
Foods that contain no animal meat or products made from animal meat.

V+ **Vegan**
Foods that contain no animal meat or animal byproducts, like eggs or honey.

VB **Varies by brand**
Check the nutrition label on the product to confirm how the product has been made.

You can create your own combinations by mixing different portion options from the swap lists, too! For example, if you're making the Greek-Style Tzatziki Chicken Wrap (page 138), you'll want to break up the protein portions to use 2 portions for chicken breast, and 1 portion for nonfat Greek yogurt to make the tzatziki sauce. Then, you can add a tortilla as your source of starch and divide 2 portions of extra-virgin olive oil as your source of healthy fats between cooking the chicken and preparing the tzatziki sauce, then fill up the wrap with non-starchy vegetables. There's no limit to how much non-starchy vegetables you can have. The more, the better!

how to build your meals

First, look at the Meal Builder for your group. Choose from the starch, protein, fat, and fruit options based on the number of portions that are indicated for each meal.

You'll see that carbohydrates are divided into starches and fruit. Starches are those foods that are traditionally referred to as carbs, like bread, pasta, and rice, as well as starchy vegetables like potatoes. They're separated into their own starch and fruit groups in your Meal Builder to guarantee that you eat a balanced variety of both sources of carbohydrate.

Similarly, you'll notice that certain starchy vegetables, like beans and chickpeas, are classified as both starch and protein due to their high protein content. The same goes for certain dairy products that you'll find in the protein and fat groups to give you more variety to choose from.

No matter which group you're in, you can add limitless non-starchy vegetables to accompany all of your meals. Veggies add essential nutrients, color, and texture to your plate. You can enjoy them any way you want to make your meals all the more satisfying! Just be mindful that when cooking veggies with oil, a teaspoon counts as one portion of fat.

FLAVOR BOOSTERS

Amp up your cooking and add nuance to food with these flavor-enhancing add-ons that won't count toward your meals.

- ketchup*
- yellow mustard
- Dijon mustard
- horseradish
- pure vanilla extract
- salsa
- garlic
- vinegar
- balsamic vinegar
- apple cider vinegar
- pickles*
- low-sodium or unsalted broths
- baking powder
- coffee
- tea
- dried herbs
- fresh herbs
- fresh lime juice
- fresh lemon juice
- low-sodium soy sauce
- coconut aminos
- tamari
- fish sauce
- Worcestershire sauce
- stevia
- Buffalo hot sauce
- sriracha sauce

Up to 7 times per week
- Unsweetened plain almond milk, 1 cup (235 ml)

Up to 7 times per week
Choose 1
- Canned crushed tomatoes, ½ cup (90 g)
- Canned diced tomatoes, ½ cup (90 g)
- Tomato paste, 2 tablespoons

Up to 4 times per week
Choose 1
- Honey, 1 tablespoon
- Maple syrup, 1 tablespoon
- Barbecue sauce, 2 tablespoons*
- Hoisin sauce, 2 tablespoons
- Teriyaki sauce, 2 tablespoons

Up to 3 times per week
- Cornstarch or arrowroot, 1 tablespoon

select a brand without added sugars

SALT

The American Heart Association's recommendation for sodium intake is no more than 2,300 milligrams per day—about one teaspoon of salt. Think of the teaspoon as your total daily budget for salt as you cook your meals. I prefer Himalayan pink salt or sea salt over regular table salt because of the coarse texture, but use any kind you want. Although some salts may be marketed as healthier options than others, they all have similar nutritional values and comparable quantities of sodium.

Certain sauces, like soy sauce, tamari, and coconut aminos, also contain sodium. For example, a tablespoon (15 ml) of low-sodium soy sauce contains about 600 mg of sodium, accounting for a quarter of the daily recommended sodium limit. Coconut aminos (which has a similar flavor to soy sauce) contains about half of that.

It's a good idea to refrain from adding salt to meals that call for one of these already-salty sauces. This is taken into account in the recipes, and most of the seasonings and sauces in this book contain no added salt to make it easier for you to control your sodium intake.

COOKING OIL

If you don't want to spend a portion of fats on oil when cooking, a good alternative is to use an extra-virgin olive oil, avocado oil, or coconut oil cooking spray instead. As long as you stick to a couple of quick sprays per meal, you don't have to take it into account in your daily total for fats.

You can also sauté completely oil-free! All you need is a good nonstick pan and low-sodium broth or water. Use a tablespoon or two (15 to 30 ml) of liquid to keep food from sticking to the pan. If you're sautéing foods with high water content, like onions or mushrooms, you won't need to add as much liquid on the pan, as these vegetables release water when they come in contact with heat.

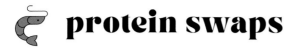

protein swaps

S	Standard	V Vegetarian
DF	Dairy-free	V+ Vegan
GF	Gluten-free	VB Varies by brand

FOOD (DAILY)	1 PORTION	SUITABILITY
Anchovies in water, drained	1 oz (30 g)	S, GF, DF
Beans, canned or cooked	¼ cup (60 g)	ALL
Canadian bacon, cooked	2 slices (1 oz [30 g])	S, GF, DF
Catfish, cooked	1½ oz (45 g)	S, GF, DF
Chicken breast, boneless and skinless, cooked	1 oz (30 g)	S, GF, DF
Chicken drumsticks, skinless, cooked	1 oz (30 g)	S, GF, DF
Chicken thighs, bone-in and skinless, cooked	1 oz (30 g)	S, GF, DF
Chickpeas, canned or cooked	¼ cup (45 g)	ALL
Clams, cooked	1 oz (30 g)	S, GF, DF
Cod, cooked	2 oz (60 g)	S, GF, DF
Cottage cheese, low-fat	⅓ cup (75 g)	S, GF, V
Crabmeat, cooked	2 oz (60 g)	S, GF, DF
Crayfish, cooked	2 oz (60 g)	S, GF, DF
Edadame, shelled	¼ cup (40 g)	ALL
Egg, small	1	S, GF, DF, V
Egg replacement	⅓ cup (75 g)	ALL
Egg whites	3	S, GF, DF, V
Greek yogurt, nonfat, plain	⅓ cup (80 ml)	S, GF, V
Ground chicken breast, cooked	1 oz (30 g)	S, GF, DF
Ground turkey (93-99%), cooked	1 oz (30 g)	S, GF, DF
Haddock, cooked	2 oz (60 g)	S, GF, DF
Lentils, cooked	¼ cup (20 g)	ALL

FOOD (DAILY)	1 PORTION	SUITABILITY
Lobster, cooked	2 oz (60 g)	S, GF, DF
Mackerel, cooked	1 oz (30 g)	S, GF, DF
Mahi-mahi, cooked	1½ oz (45 g)	S, GF, DF
Meatless soy crumbles	⅓ cup (45 g)	ALL
Milk, skim	½ cup (120 ml)	S, GF, V
Mozzarella cheese, fat-free	¼ cup shredded (1 oz [30 g])	S, GF, V
Nutritional yeast	2 tbsp	ALL
Octopus or squid, cooked	1 oz (30 g)	S, GF, DF
Oysters, cooked	2 oz (60 g)	S, GF, DF
Pollock, cooked	1½ oz (45 g)	S, GF, DF
Protein powder	1 tbsp	VB
Quark, nonfat, plain	⅓ cup (65 g)	S, GF, V
Salmon, cooked	1 oz (30 g)	S, GF, DF
Sardines in water, drained	1 oz (30 g)	S, GF, DF
Scallops, cooked	1½ oz (45 g)	S, GF, DF
Sea bass, cooked	1½ oz (45 g)	S, GF, DF
Seitan	1 thin slice (1 oz [30 g])	ALL
Shrimp, cooked	2 oz (60 g)	S, GF, DF
Smoked salmon	1 oz (30 g)	S, GF, DF
Snapper, cooked	1½ oz (45 g)	S, GF, DF
Soy milk, unsweetened, plain	1 cup (235 ml)	VB
Swiss cheese, low-fat	¼ cup shredded (1 oz [30 g])	S, GF, V

FOOD (ENJOY UP TO 3 TIMES/WEEK)	1 PORTION	SUITABILITY
Bacon, cooked	1 slice (¼ oz [8 g])	S, GF, DF
Blue cheese, reduced fat	3 tbsp crumbled (¾ oz [20 g])	S, GF, V
Cheddar cheese, shredded	2 tbsp (½ oz [15 g])	S, GF, V
Chorizo sausage	½ oz (15 g)	S, GF, DF
Colby cheese, reduced fat	¾ oz (20 g)	S, GF, V
Feta cheese, reduced fat	3 tbsp crumbled (¾ oz [20 g])	S, GF, V
Gouda cheese	½ oz (15 g)	S, GF, V
Greek yogurt, low-fat, plain	⅓ cup (80 ml)	S, GF, V
Greek yogurt, low-fat, vanilla	¼ cup (60 ml)	S, GF, V
Greek yogurt, nonfat, vanilla	⅓ cup (80 ml)	S, GF, V
Ground beef (95%), cooked	1 oz (30 g)	S, GF, DF
Ham, deli sliced, lean	1½ slices (1½ oz [45 g])	S, GF, DF
Lamb rib chops, trimmed, cooked	1 oz (30 g)	S, GF, DF
Mexican-style cheese, reduced fat	3 tbsp shredded (¾ oz [20 g])	S, GF, V

FOOD (ENJOY UP TO 3 TIMES/WEEK)	1 PORTION	SUITABILITY
Mozzarella cheese, part-skim	2 tbsp shredded (½ oz [15 g])	S, GF, V
Parmesan cheese, grated	2 tbsp (½ oz [15 g])	S, GF, V
Pork chops, lean and trimmed, cooked	1 oz (30 g)	S, GF, DF
Pork tenderloin, lean, cooked	1 oz (30 g)	S, GF, DF
Provolone cheese	½ oz (15 g)	S, GF, V
Provolone cheese, reduced fat	¾ oz (20 g)	S, GF, V
Ricotta cheese, part-skim	1 oz (30 g)	S, GF, V
Romano cheese, grated	2 tbsp (½ oz [15 g])	S, GF, V
Steak, lean, cooked	1 oz (30 g)	S, GF, DF
Sweet Italian sausage	1 oz (30 g)	S, GF, DF
Swiss cheese	2 tbsp shredded (½ oz [15 g])	S, GF, V
Yogurt, lowfat, plain	⅓ cup (80 ml)	S, GF, V
Yogurt, lowfat, vanilla	¼ cup (60 ml)	S, GF, V
Yogurt, nonfat, vanilla	¼ cup (60 ml)	S, GF, V

For information on uncooked weights for meat, poultry, and seafood, see page 79.

FOOD (DAILY)	1 PORTION	SUITABILITY
wordfish, cooked	1 oz (30 g)	S, GF, DF
empeh	1 slice (1 oz [30 g])	ALL
extured soy	2 tbsp	ALL
ilapia, cooked	1½ oz (45 g)	S, GF, DF
ofu, firm or extra firm	2 oz (60 g)	ALL
ofu, silken or soft	3 oz (85 g)	ALL
rout, cooked	1 oz (30 g)	S, GF, DF
una in oil, drained	1 oz (30 g)	S, GF, DF
una in water, drained	2 oz (60 g)	S, GF, DF
urkey breast, cooked	1 oz (30 g)	S, GF, DF
urkey breast, deli sliced	2 slices (1 oz [30 g])	S, GF, DF
urkey bacon, cooked	2 slices (1 oz [30 g])	S, GF, DF
hitefish, cooked	1 oz (30 g)	S, GF, DF
ogurt, nonfat, plain	⅓ cup (80 ml)	S, GF, V

unlimited non-starchy vegetables

lfafa sprouts	Chinese cabbage	Onions
rtichoke	Chinese spinach	Peppers
rugula	Coleslaw	Radicchio
sparagus	Collard greens	Radishes
amboo shoots	Cucumber	Romaine lettuce
ean sprouts	Eggplant	Scallions
eets	Fennel	Shallots
ell peppers	Garlic	Spinach
ok choy	Green beans	Sprouts
russels sprouts	Hearts of palm	Swiss chard
roccoli	Herbs	Tomatillos
abbage	Jicama	Tomatoes
auliflower	Kale	Turnips
arrots	Leeks	Water chestnuts
elery	Lettuce	Watercress
hayote	Mushrooms	Zucchini
hicory	Okra	

🍉 fruit swaps

FOOD (DAILY)	1 PORTION	SUITABILITY
Apple	1 small	ALL
Apricot	3 medium	ALL
Banana	½ small	ALL
Blackberries	¾ cup (100 g)	ALL
Blueberries	½ cup (70 g)	ALL
Cherries	¾ cup (85 g)	ALL
Coconut water	1 cup (235 ml)	ALL
Cranberries	1 cup (100 g)	ALL
Dates	2	ALL
Dragon fruit	1 medium	ALL
Grapefruit	1 small	ALL
Grapes	½ cup (70 g)	ALL
Guava	½ cup (85 g)	ALL
Honeydew melon	1 cup (175 g)	ALL
Jackfruit	⅓ cup (50 g)	ALL
Kiwi	1 medium	ALL
Lemon	Untracked	ALL
Lime	Untracked	ALL
Mamey sapote	¼ cup (45 g)	ALL
Mango	½ cup (85 g)	ALL
Mixed berries	½ cup (85 g)	ALL
Nectarine	1 small	ALL
Orange	1 small	ALL
Papaya	½ cup (100 g)	ALL
Passion fruit	3	ALL
Peach	1 small	ALL
Pear	½ small	ALL
Pineapple	½ cup (85 g)	ALL
Plums	1 large	ALL
Pomegranate seeds	⅓ cup (55 g)	ALL
Raisins	2 tbsp	ALL
Raspberries	¾ cup (100 g)	ALL
Strawberries	1 cup (140 g)	ALL
Tangerines	1 medium	ALL
Watermelon	1 cup (140 g)	ALL

FOOD (ENJOY UP TO ONCE A WEEK)	1 PORTION	SUITABILITY
Applesauce, unsweetened	½ cup (120 ml)	ALL
Dried fruit mix	2 tbsp	ALL
Orange juice, freshly squeezed	½ cup (120 ml)	ALL
Raisins	2 tbsp	ALL

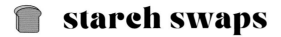

starch swaps

S	Standard	V	Vegetarian
DF	Dairy-free	V+	Vegan
GF	Gluten-free	VB	Varies by brand

FOOD (DAILY)	1 PORTION	SUITABILITY
Acorn squash, cooked	½ medium (160 g)	ALL
Amaranth, cooked	⅓ cup (80 g)	ALL
Baby corn, fresh	1½ cup (200 g)	ALL
Baby potatoes	1 cup (85 g)	ALL
Beans, canned or cooked	½ cup (115 g)	ALL
Brown rice, cooked	½ cup (100 g)	ALL
Brown rice pasta, cooked	½ cup (30 g)	ALL
Buckwheat (soba) noodles, cooked	¾ cup (85 g)	ALL
Bulgur, cooked	½ cup (90 g)	S, DF, V, V+
Butternut squash	1 cup (200 g)	ALL
Cereal, unsweetened	½ cup (15 g)	VB
Cellophane noodles, dry	1 oz (30 g)	ALL
Chestnuts	¾ cup (100 g)	ALL
Chickpea pasta, cooked	⅔ cup (55 g)	VB
Chickpeas, canned or cooked	⅓ cup (55 g)	ALL
Coconut flour	3 tbsp (20 g)	ALL
Corn, canned or cooked	⅔ cup (110 g)	ALL
Cornmeal	3 tbsp (30 g)	ALL
Corn tortillas, 4" (10 cm)	2 (1 oz [30 g])	ALL
Couscous, cooked	½ cup (85 g)	VB
Egg noodles, cooked	½ cup (80 g)	VB
Freekeh, cooked	½ cup (120 g)	S, DF, V, V+
Gluten-free bread	1 slice (1 oz [30 g])	VB
Green peas	¾ cup (100 g)	ALL
Gluten-free pasta	½ cup (70 g)	VB
Grits, cooked	½ cup (130 g)	ALL
Lentil pasta, cooked	⅔ cup (135 g)	ALL
Lentils, cooked	½ cup (40 g)	ALL
Malanga, cooked	½ cup (65 g)	ALL
Millet, cooked	½ cup (85 g)	ALL
Oatmilk, unsweetened	1 cup (235 ml)	VB

FOOD (DAILY)	1 PORTION	SUITABILITY
Pea pasta, cooked	½ cup (100 g)	VB
Pearled barley, cooked	½ cup (80 g)	S, DF, V, V+
Pidgeon peas (gandules), cooked	½ cup (165 g)	ALL
Plantains	½ medium (90 g)	ALL
Popcorn, air popped	3 cups (25 g)	ALL
Pumpkin, cooked	2 cups (490 g)	ALL
Pumpkin, pureed	1 cup (225 g)	ALL
Quinoa, cooked	½ cup (95 g)	ALL
Red potato, cooked	1 small (3½ oz [100 g])	ALL
Refried beans, canned	½ cup (125 g)	VB
Rice cakes	3 (1 oz [30 g])	VB
Rice milk	¾ cup (175 ml)	ALL
Rice paper wrappers	3 (1¾ oz [50 g])	ALL
Rolled oats, old fashioned	⅓ cup (1 oz [30 g])	ALL
Snow peas	1½ cups (100 g)	ALL
Spelt, cooked	⅓ cup (65 g)	S, DF, V, V+
Spelt flour tortilla, 6" (15 cm)	1 (1 oz [30 g])	VB
Sprouted grain bread	1 slice (1 oz [30 g])	S, DF, V, V+
Sweet potato, cooked	1 small (4 oz [115 g])	ALL
Thin rye crispbreads	3 (1 oz [30 g])	S, DF, V, V+
White potato, cooked	1 small (3½ oz [100 g])	ALL
Whole wheat bagel	⅓ bagel (1 oz [30 g])	VB
Whole grain bread	1 slice (1 oz [30 g])	VB
Whole grain tortilla, 6" (15 cm)	1 (1 oz [30 g])	VB
Whole wheat English muffin	1 (1 oz [30 g])	VB
Whole wheat pita bread, small (4" [10 cm] pitette)	1 (1 oz [30 g])	S, DF, V, V+
Whole wheat spaghetti, cooked	½ cup (70 g)	VB
Wild rice, cooked	½ cup (80 g)	ALL
Yucca, cooked	⅓ cup (1½ oz [45 g])	ALL

FOOD (ENJOY UP TO 3 TIMES/WEEK)	1 PORTION	SUITABILITY
Bagel, plain	⅓ bagel (1 oz [30 g])	VB
Burger bun	½ bun (1 oz [30 g])	VB
Buttermilk, low-fat	1 cup (235 ml)	S, GF, V
Corn flakes	1 cup (1 oz [30 g])	VB
Croutons	⅓ cup (1 oz [30 g])	VB
English muffin	½ muffin ((1 oz [30 g])	VB
Flour tortilla, 6" (15 cm)	1 small (1 oz [30 g])	VB
Granola	¼ cup (1 oz [30 g])	VB

FOOD (ENJOY UP TO 3 TIMES/WEEK)	1 PORTION	SUITABILITY
Greek yogurt, whole milk	½ cup (120 ml)	S, GF, V
Milk, whole	⅔ cup (160 ml)	S, GF, V
Pasta, regular, cooked	½ cup (100 g)	VB
Ramen noodles, dry	1 oz (30 g)	VB
Rice flour	2 tbsp	ALL
White pita bread, small (4" [10 cm] pitette)	1 (1 oz [30 g])	S, DF, V, V+
White rice, cooked	½ cup (90 g)	ALL
Yogurt, whole milk	⅔ cup (160 ml)	S, GF, V

fat swaps

FOOD (DAILY)	1 PORTION	SUITABILITY
Almond milk yogurt, plain, unsweetened	¼ cup (60 ml)	ALL
Avocado	¼ small (1 oz [30 g])	ALL
Avocado oil	1 tsp	ALL
Almond butter	½ tbsp	ALL
Almond flour	1 tbsp	ALL
Almonds	1½ tbsp	ALL
Brazil nuts	1 tbsp	ALL
Cacao nibs	1 tbsp	ALL
Cacao powder	2 tbsp	ALL
Cashew butter	½ tbsp	ALL
Cashews	1 tbsp	ALL
Chia seeds	1 tbsp	ALL
Chimichurri sauce	1 tbsp	ALL
Egg, small	1	S, GF, DF, V
Extra-virgin olive oil	1 tsp	ALL

FOOD (DAILY)	1 PORTION	SUITABILITY
Flaxseeds	1 tbsp	ALL
Guacamole	2 tbsp	ALL
Hazelnuts	1 tbsp	ALL
Mayonnaise, low-fat	1 tbsp	S, GF, V
Olives	8	ALL
Peanut butter	½ tbsp	ALL
Peanuts	1 tbsp	ALL
Pecans, chopped	1 tbsp	ALL
Pesto sauce	½ tbsp	ALL
Pistachios	1 tbsp	ALL
Sesame oil	1 tsp	ALL
Sesame seeds	1 tbsp	ALL
Sunflower seeds	1 tbsp	ALL
Tahini	1 tsp	ALL
Walnuts, chopped	1 tbsp	ALL

FOOD (ENJOY UP TO 3 TIMES/WEEK)	1 PORTION	SUITABILITY
Blue cheese	2 tbsp crumbled (½ oz [15 g])	S, GF, V
Blue cheese, reduced fat	3 tbsp crumbled (¾ oz [20 g])	S, GF, V
Butter, unsalted	½ tbsp	S, GF, V
Cheddar cheese	2 tbsp (½ oz [15 g])	S, GF, V
Coconut, fresh, sliced	2 tbsp	ALL
Coconut cream, canned, unsweetened	1 tbsp	ALL
Coconut milk, canned, unsweetened	2 tbsp	ALL
Coconut oil	1 tsp	ALL
Colby cheese	½ oz (15 g)	S, GF, V
Colby cheese, reduced fat	¾ oz (20 g)	S, GF, V
Cream cheese spread, low fat	1 tbsp	S, GF, V
Dark chocolate chips	½ tbsp	VB
Feta cheese	2 tbsp crumbled (½ oz [15 g])	S, GF, V
Feta cheese, reduced fat	3 tbsp crumbled (¾ oz [20 g])	S, GF, V
Goat cheese	2 tbsp crumbled (½ oz [15 g])	S, GF, V

FOOD (ENJOY UP TO 3 TIMES/WEEK)	1 PORTION	SUITABILITY
Goat cheese, reduced fat	¼ cup crumbled (1 oz [30 g])	S, GF, V
Gouda cheese	½ oz (15 g)	S, GF, V
Mexican-style cheese, reduced fat	3 tbsp shredded (¾ oz [20 g])	S, GF, V
Mozzarella cheese, part-skim	2 tbsp shredded (½ oz [15 g])	S, GF, V
Nutella spread	½ tbsp	S, GF, V
Parmesan cheese, grated	2 tbsp (½ oz [15 g])	S, GF, V
Pepper jack cheese, reduced fat	2 tbsp shredded (¾ oz [20 g])	S, GF, V
Plant-based cheese shreds	2 tbsp	ALL
Provolone cheese	½ oz (15 g)	S, GF, V
Provolone cheese, reduced fat	¾ oz (20 g)	S, GF, V
Romano cheese, grated	2 tbsp (½ oz [15 g])	S, GF, V
Sour cream, reduced fat	2 tbsp	S, GF, V
Swiss cheese	2 tbsp shredded (½ oz [15 g])	S, GF, V
Shredded coconut, unsweetened	2 tbsp	ALL

SAUCES

Sauces are a fantastic way to add flavor to your foods and tie a meal together! To make a tomato-based sauce, use canned crushed or diced tomatoes. Both are on the flavor booster list, and you can have half a cup per day without it counting toward your meals. For a creamy white sauce, my preferred method is to use 1 cup (235 ml) of plain unsweetened almond milk with a tablespoon-ish (15 ml) of low-sodium soy sauce as a base. Then mix it with sautéed garlic, onion, mushroom, or any other vegetables you love to have in your white sauce, plus herbs and spices. Finally, add a tablespoon (8 g) of cornstarch or arrowroot mixed with water as a slurry to thicken the sauce. Recipes for flavorful spice mixes and seasonings start on page 84.

BEVERAGES

Most of us require between 70 and 100 ounces (2 to 3 L) of water per day. If you struggle to meet your water goal, mealtimes are a great opportunity to boost your intake. We often assume that if we feel normal, we're staying hydrated enough, but are we really? To find out, try measuring your personal water goal (which we calculated on page 53) into a large bottle at night and stash it in the fridge, so you'll have ice cold water to enjoy the following day. If you have some left at night, you'll know how much more you need to drink to meet your goal.

If you like your tea sweet, use stevia or honey as a sweetener instead of sugar. And if you enjoy your coffee with milk, try swapping cow's milk with plain, unsweetened almond milk. Just be mindful of your caffeine intake—although caffeine sensitivity can vary per person, for most healthy adults, up to 400 mg of caffeine per day is considered safe. For reference, 400 mg per day can mean four to five brewed coffees or six shots of espresso. But if you don't need that much, less is always better! For more refreshing drink inspiration, check out the fruity beverages on pages 195–197.

meal builder q&a

Can I switch meals around or combine two meals while at work? As long as you eat all five meals, feel free to rearrange them in a way that works best for you. While I highly encourage you to eat every three to four hours to help curb cravings and avoid getting hungry in the middle of the day, I understand there can be times when it is simply not possible. If your mornings are busy, pick an AM snack that is easy to pack with you to work and have on your desk, or on the go. If keeping regular mealtimes at work is a challenge, you may combine breakfast, lunch, or dinner with the AM or PM snack from your Meal Builder and have your remaining three meals at their regular times.

Can I remove a portion from one meal and add it to another one? Yes! Your meals are planned to maximize balance and variety, but you can consider them suggestions rather than strict rules. You can move portions around and use them as rollovers for another meal if you feel like it. I do this all the time depending on what I'm in the mood for; I think of my portions for the day as a total budget that I work within. For example, you can take half a portion of starch from lunch and add it for a larger dinner, or you can have two portions of fruit with your PM snack by borrowing a fruit portion from breakfast. Or, if you're craving dark chocolate chips or shredded coconut in your PM snack, you can borrow a portion of fat from another meal.

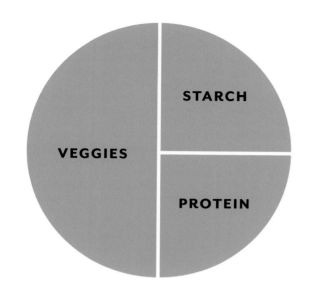

What if I didn't follow my Meal Builder for a meal? Be kind to yourself and remember that this is a lifestyle, not a temporary fix. One meal or treat won't derail you from your path or hurt your progress! I encourage you to enjoy the memories created on special events like birthdays or a dinner out with friends. The program focuses on the big picture. Being able to enjoy any meal without deprivation or guilt is where long-lasting change happens. Plus, attempting to completely cut out what we love often leads to eating even more. Don't try to compensate by eating less or exercising more than you normally would to make up for it; simply move on and return to eating within the guidelines again for your next meal. If you feel you need more work on establishing a positive relationship with food, you can always check back to chapter 3!

Can I ever eat out if I want to stay on track with my eating? If it's for a special occasion, focus on enjoying yourself rather than stressing about your food choices. Carry on with your regular meals before and after eating out. If you eat out often because of work or other commitments, select an option from the menu that best fits your Meal Builder, even if it's not a perfect match. Ask for a healthier swap if you can't find what you're looking for. Limit creamy dressings and sauces. Choose water as your beverage. Keep protein powder on you for a quick shake after your meal for those times when a restaurant had a poor selection of options.

If the restaurant allows you to customize your meal, or if you go to a salad bar where you can build the plate yourself, aim to follow this easy model:

½ **OF THE PLATE:** fresh or steamed vegetables

¼ **OF THE PLATE:** lean proteins, such as a filet of grilled chicken or fish

¼ **OF THE PLATE:** starches, such as rice or baked potato

Can I mix different orange foods from the food swap lists? Yes, as long as you select those foods applying the guidelines. Note that the guidelines apply per meal, rather than per portion. For example, if you are meal prepping two steak bowls for the same week, and you eat one with brown rice and the other with white rice, you'll have one more meal left to enjoy any item from the orange foods list for protein, and two for starch. You may need to use more than one item from one food group's orange list to cook a dish or mix items from the lists for different food groups, and that's fine. Remember that these items are not "bad" foods! As we saw in the previous chapters, certain foods come with guidelines to ensure that your meals are nutritious and as beneficial as possible to your health. While their calorie content is similar, the swap tables consider other nutritional factors, like added sugars, fiber, and saturated fats versus unsaturated fats.

What if I'm used to eating less food? Eating five times a day may seem like a lot of food if you haven't had structured mealtimes before, if you've eaten less frequently with a lower protein or fiber intake, or if you've been on very restrictive calorie diets prior to this program. I understand—I've been there myself! But your *Sculpt* meals have been designed carefully to give you the energy to power through the day and exercise, while helping you burn fat at optimal levels at every group level. If you're finding it difficult to finish your meals, I recommend choosing smoothies or shakes that can feel less voluminous than solid food, rather than skipping a meal. You may find that as you progress through your program, your appetite increases as your metabolism speeds up.

What if I'm used to eating more food? You should feel satisfied but not stuffed after finishing a meal. If your meals feel small, load up your plate with more non-starchy vegetables. They are filled with nutrients like vitamins, potassium, and fiber, which will help you stay full. If you still feel you aren't happy with the amount of food, or if you recently switched groups and you're not yet used to the new amounts, you may add an extra portion of fat or protein to your day for one week, and then continue with the regular Meal Builder meals for your group.

Do I need to modify my meals if I work in shifts or have a very irregular schedule? If you have extended hours in a day, your mealtimes will remain the same by eating every three to four hours. If you're required to stay up more hours than average, start your first meal by eating within thirty minutes from the time you wake up and proceed with extra snacks (choose between AM and PM snack) every three to four hours until you go to sleep, even when it exceeds the five mealtimes per day. Because you will be up longer, you'll need the extra energy from food. If you have an irregular schedule, prepping your meals ahead of time will make all the difference in simplifying your days!

Should I switch meals around my workouts? If you work out intensely in the morning, switch your meals around so you can have lunch as a post-workout meal to ensure that you get plenty of carbohydrates and protein for recovery. The same applies if you exercise in the evening: Dinner should be your post-workout meal.

What if I'm not used to measuring my portions? The program uses a kitchen scale and measuring cups and spoons as tools to make it easier to build your meals and get familiar with healthy meal sizes. Because the portions are worked out for you, all you need to do is measure the ingredients you select.

Think about it like this: with enough repetition, your brain learns to recognize what beneficial portions look like, until putting them together feels like second nature. It shifts you from eating on autopilot to eating with awareness. We certainly won't ask you to keep measuring your portions forever. But it's an effective way to get used to grasping what your portions should look like until you've become so familiar with the program that you can confidently take a step toward an intuitive eating approach. At first, it's essential, unless you are experienced with what an ounce of cooked chicken breast or two ounces of dry pasta look like. Measuring is highly recommended over guesstimating when it comes to portions. Underestimating often leads to oversized portions, which can be a major contributor to weight gain.

Are any of the portions interchangeable?

Your Meal Builder is designed with an ideal macronutrient distribution to support you in feeling great, productive, and energized all day. It is recommended that you stick to the meal structure to your best ability to ensure that you're getting optimal quantities of nutrients from every food group. But if you want to make an occasional adjustment, you can swap one portion of protein, fat, or fruit interchangeably, or either one of those portions with half a portion of starch.

Do I have to include fruit portions in meals? You can,
or you can incorporate fresh fruit as dessert. Fruit is a great way to get your fiber fix and immune-strengthening antioxidants, and you'll also find multiple recipes with fruit included in the ingredient lists.

What if I'm not used to eating vegetables?

There are so many ways to incorporate vegetables into your meals. You don't have to eat vegetables that you dislike, or any foods for that matter! You can start by including veggies in your smoothies, pasta sauces, sandwiches, or wraps. Try them raw, sautéed, steamed, or roasted! Start small—a handful of spinach in a berry smoothie, sautéed broccoli and mushrooms in pasta sauce, or some onion and celery in a stew or soup. As you get used to the taste, gradually keep adding more.

How can I transition to Sculpt if I've been on
a low-carb diet for a long time? Begin by choosing your starch portions from the green list. They take longer to digest and won't cause major blood sugar spikes like some of the simple carbs included in the orange list. Focusing on the quality of your carbohydrate sources makes a significant difference when transitioning to a balanced approach from a very low-carb diet. It's important to know that when you incorporate more carbohydrates again, your weight will probably go up a few pounds at first. This occurs because the body naturally pulls water with each gram of glycogen it stores as energy from carbohydrates you eat. Usually, it takes about one to two weeks for the body to adjust fully, depending on how restricted your diet was before starting the program.

unlocking your kitchen confidence

FOOD IS FUEL. It's also a big part of family life, cultural celebrations, and so much more. Too often, as we rush through the day marking things off our endless to-do lists, we dedicate the bare minimum of our time to preparing proper meals, and that often ends up taking a toll on our health and weight.

Wellness starts in the kitchen. Making the most of your meals at home is crucial to the success of your transition toward a healthier, happier life. While home-cooked meals require some planning, they make losing weight (not to mention life!) a lot easier.

In this chapter, I will show you:

- timesaving meal prep strategies
- various meal prep methods
- cooking and storage tips for easy everyday meals
- how to boost flavors with herbs and spices

If you're anything like the old me, the idea of cooking all your meals from scratch may sound next to impossible. Getting dinner on the table every day is no small feat when paired with a hectic life. We're all busy and tired by the time we get home. Between work, school, kids, pets, laundry . . . who really has the time to cook, let alone make healthy meals?

I had those same concerns until I discovered something that changed my life. Yep, you guessed it—meal prep. With your Meal Builder and this chapter's meal planning template, you've got all the tools you need to make the seemingly overwhelming totally achievable. Knowing what to eat is a great start, but having a plan in place so you actually have those foods available and avoid rushed decisions? Even better.

here's to fuss-free cooking

Trust me when I say that meal planning is one of the most beneficial habits you can build for yourself. It doesn't sound glamorous, but when you commit to a better lifestyle, you'll want to have more control over what goes on your plate. It makes you the boss of your food choices.

And cooking can be so much more than a task. Once you get into it, it can become a self-care ritual that you look forward to. And that is when the *Sculpt* way of eating becomes a lifestyle you'll want to keep up forever and never look back.

Meal prepping puts you in control of what you eat and helps you manage your portions better. But believe

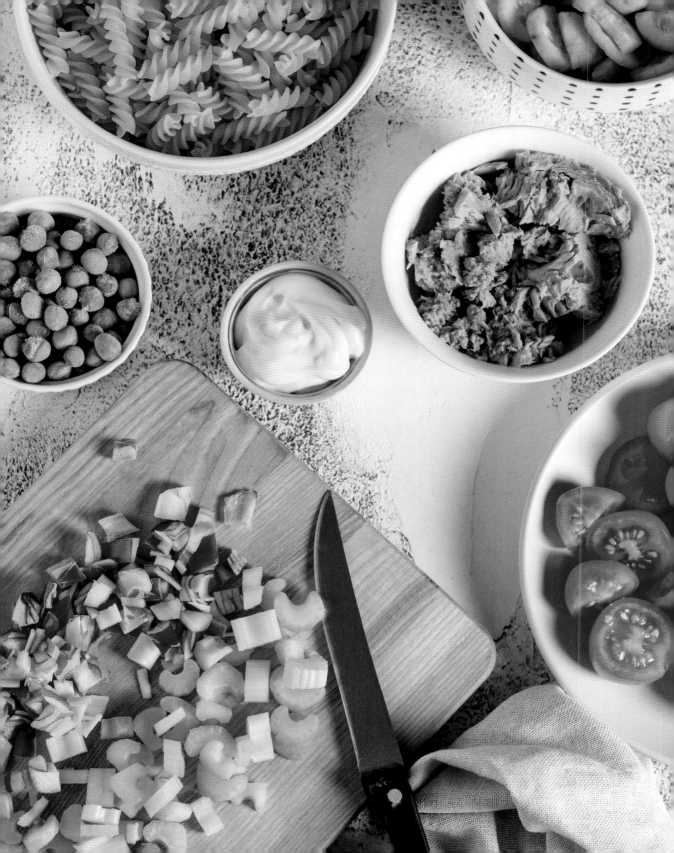

it or not, it's a killer life strategy, too. Yes, it takes some up-front effort, but it saves you a ton of work on weekdays. It guarantees that you always have healthy options at your fingertips, minimizing situations where you may have previously picked up takeout or made your way to a drive-through. And meal prep is way more cost-effective than eating out, so you'll be saving a lot of money and also reducing food waste.

And here's the real truth bomb: Healthy eating does not have to be complicated. You don't need to make a fuss or use any elaborate cooking techniques to make healthy, flavorful meals. Changing up cooking styles helps expand your culinary skills and find new favorite dishes to enjoy. Tired of pan-cooked chicken? Try poaching, air frying, slow cooking, baking, or grilling it. Marinate it, try new sauces, or pair it with a different side. Spice things up and experiment with flavor combinations and seasoning blends later in this chapter until you feel comfortable to improvise on your own. Plus, your time in the kitchen doesn't have to be boring—make it fun! Put on music or catch up on your favorite podcast while cooking.

GETTING ORGANIZED

An organized kitchen is the foundation of quick-and-easy cooking. Keep your kitchen clean and decluttered, and you won't have to spend time searching for every tool and ingredient. Revamp your kitchen to create easy access to tools. Clean out your pantry, fridge, and freezer so you have room to store your containers. Expired condiments, forgotten leftovers, and questionable produce all belong in the trash. When you're finished, you'll feel more at ease and ready to start the program.

I prepare for the week ahead by buying groceries and prepping most of my meals during the weekend.

It has become a ritual for me every Sunday! If Sunday isn't convenient for you, pick any other day that best suits your schedule.

As an alternative to the traditional one-day-a-week meal prep method, you can divide your meal prep between two days of the week based on the type of dishes you'll be making. I do my grocery shopping just once a week, but I prefer to add a second meal prep day to my week whenever my schedule allows it. A second day helps to ensure that your meals taste fresher. If you've ever had grilled chicken that's been sitting in the fridge for more than a couple of days, you'll get what I mean!

And because convenience is king, I try to plan my food choices and select my meal prep method for the week based on what my calendar looks like. To help me plan better, I use the meal prep planner that I've shared with you on the next page.

METHOD #1: MEAL PREP ONCE PER WEEK

This method makes the most of your time, and it can be a huge help in reducing decision fatigue. It is the ideal choice if you make recipes that call for cooking all the ingredients in the same pan, pot, cooker, or sheet pan. If you own a slow cooker, I encourage you to put it to use with this method of meal prep—just load in all the ingredients before bed, let it cook overnight, and wake up to amazing tasting food!

For meals that you won't be cooking on the actual meal prep day, pre-prep dry ingredients, excluding any liquids, and place them into airtight meal prep containers or freezer bags for each recipe you'll be making in the week. Label them and pop them in the fridge or freezer to speed up the process when you cook them. When it comes to convenience, that's always going to be a yes in my book!

meal prep planner

Circle the day(s) when you know you'll realistically have time to dedicate to meal prep:

S   M   T   W   T   F   S

How much time will you have for meal prepping each day? _____

Circle the day(s) when you'll do your grocery shopping, or schedule groceries to be delivered:

S   M   T   W   T   F   S

Choose the day(s) that the first meal prep day will cover:

S   M   T   W   T   F   S

Entire week

Choose the meals that you'll be prepping on the first meal prep day:

Breakfast   PM snack
AM snack   Dinner
Lunch   All meals

Choose the day(s) that the second meal prep day will cover (optional):

S   M   T   W   T   F   S

Entire week

Choose the meals that you'll be prepping on the second meal prep day (optional):

Breakfast   PM snack
AM snack   Dinner
Lunch   All meals

Using your group's Meal Builder and recipes, write down what you'll make for each meal of the week. This includes make-ahead and same-day meals. Check the fridge, freezer, and pantry. What ingredients (if any) do you need to buy?

Day	Breakfast	AM Snack	Lunch	PM Snack	Dinner
Monday					
Tuesday					
Wednesday					
Thursday					
Friday					
Saturday					
Sunday					

METHOD #2: MEAL PREP TWICE PER WEEK

If you prefer ready-to-eat, reheatable meal kits, or you're an adventurous eater who enjoys having wiggle room when it comes to eating, prepping meals twice a week might work better for you. It will still be much more efficient than preparing food from scratch every night. To maximize variety throughout the week, make batches of the basics: Cook grains, proteins, and vegetables, then seal and store them in separate containers.

For example, if you make three chicken breasts, place them in their own container. Do the same for fresh, roasted, or sautéed vegetables, and cooked grains. Label the container or bag so you can easily combine meal components between containers during the week. For animal proteins, like chicken and fish, squeezing in a second day of cooking during the week will ensure that your meals maintain freshness and always taste amazing.

mix up your meal prep

Big Batch Mix 'n' Match

This is the perfect way to go if you want to minimize repetition during the week. With this approach, you batch-cook each element individually. You'll store your grilled chicken in one container, roasted broccoli in another, and so on. Each day, you can easily grab what you want to eat from the fridge to prepare any meals you dream up in the week. One day, you can pair your prepped steak with asparagus and brown rice. The next day, you can choose salmon and sweet potatoes over a bed of greens.

Ready-to-Eat Meal Kits

Portioning entire precooked meals into individual containers is a great option when you know you're going to be extra pressed with time. You do all the prep and cooking on designated meal prep days. Then

To make cooking even more straightforward, recipes are marked with these icons:

 EASY & QUICK PREP Requires minimal effort and amount of prep time

 MEAL PREP FAVORITE Ideal for meal prepping and can be stored in the fridge or freezer after cooking

 NO COOK RECIPE No cooking required to make the recipe

 FAMILY FAVORITE Kid-friendly and great for the whole family to enjoy

 ONE-PAN RECIPE Combines all ingredients in one dish while cooking

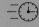 **UNDER 15 MINUTES** Takes under 15 minutes to prep and cook

each day of the week, you simply pop it in the microwave or oven to reheat when necessary. To avoid recipes with a sauce from becoming mushy in the fridge, store sauces in a separate container to toss in before serving. As a rule of thumb, unless you're making a one-pot dish, like a soup or a stew, keep wet ingredients separate from dry ingredients and combine only when you're ready to eat.

Ready-to-Cook Containers

The third way of meal prepping is great for meals like stews, soups, and smoothies. For soups and stews, portion all the dry ingredients into a bag. Freeze or refrigerate until you're ready to cook over the stove, slow cooker, pressure cooker, pan, or pot. For smoothies, pre-portion your fruits and veggies, and then freeze them. When you're ready to serve, just add the contents of the bag with water or milk, then blend and enjoy!

10 golden rules for reaching your meal prep potential

1   **Start your planning by reviewing your current group's Meal Builder.** What do the portions of your meals look like? When I'm not feeling too inspired, I like to browse through the recipes. Write down any potential changes you may want to make to the recipes you've selected with the help of swap tables. None of the recipes in this book are very challenging, but if you're new to cooking, I suggest starting simple. Try recipes marked with ⤬ and use ingredients you're familiar with. Check your pantry, fridge, and freezer to see what you already have on hand. Planning also creates a great opportunity to include any leftover ingredients!

2   **How many times have you bought food that didn't end up getting used?** Or you got home and realized that you forgot an essential ingredient for a recipe you had been wanting to try? Make a list of the ingredients you need, whether you're shopping in a physical store or ordering groceries online. Try to get your groceries either on the same day or the day before your main meal prep day to make sure nothing spoils before you can cook it.

3   **If you're using frozen meat to be cooked in the oven or slow cooker,** thaw it in the fridge overnight. If you use a pressure cooker, you can usually throw it in while it's still frozen. Just double-check your appliance's instructions before cooking. Did you know you don't have to defrost frozen vegetables? Just pour them out of the bag and cook them!

4   **If a recipe calls for sautéing, do that first,** and store the sautéed ingredients in the fridge or freezer. Only combine sautéed ingredients with the rest of the meal when you're ready to eat! Sautéed veggies will last three to four days in the fridge, but they'll be in their prime during the first couple of days.

5   **Pre-prep vegetables and fruit by washing,** drying, peeling, deseeding, trimming when appropriate, and chopping them. To go the extra mile, try making a habit out of this as soon as you get home from the grocery store or have them delivered. Prepack greens and fruit for smoothies and make pre-portioned snack bags with veggie or fruit sticks. Break broccoli and cauliflower down to have the florets ready.

6   **Try cooking certain foods in larger batches** and storing some of it in the freezer. Your future self will thank you! Most foods last three to five days in the fridge and two to three months in the freezer—use the food storage table on page 78 for reference. Whether cooking for the family, preparing for a get-together, or making batches of food to freeze, simply multiply the quantities of a recipe by the number of meals you want to make. Multiply by two to double, three to triple, and so forth. When cooking in batches, make sure you increase the quantities for all ingredients equally, so the servings can be portioned according to the Meal Builder of your group.

7 **Recognize the limits of meal prep.** Certain foods, like avocados and apples, can turn brown if prepped too far in advance. Aim to slice them no more than two to three hours before serving. If you need to get them ready earlier, store apples in cold water in an airtight container to prevent oxidation. To keep avocado from browning, keep the pit in and gently brush the flesh with lemon juice before storing. The acid in citrus helps prevent browning, but you'll also need to cover it tightly to reduce exposure to oxygen. Salads with dressing mixed in and assembled sandwiches can turn soggy in the fridge. Keep them fresh by storing dressings, spreads, or sauces in a container of their own, and then combine them upon serving.

8 **Gather recipes that have similar ingredients** cooked at the same temperatures and cook them at the same time. Start with foods that require the longest cooking time—usually this entails roasting ingredients in the oven and boiling grains like rice, quinoa, or lentils. As these ingredients are cooking, get the next part of the recipes ready.

9 **When whipping up your meals,** be careful not to overcook them. Keep in mind that reheating will cause foods to cook more and some foods, like chicken, can become extra dry if overheated already during the meal prep process.

10 **Always save whatever doesn't require heat,** like sauces, dressing, or chopping raw veggies for last! Let hot food cool after you've placed it in containers before closing the lid and storing them. Label all your containers and bags with the name of the food they contain. If you're cooking meal kits from recipes, mark them with the recipe name and cooking date. Make a note of anything that isn't included during meal prep with directions on what to add later.

HOW LONG CAN I STORE FOOD?

Food	Fridge life	Freezer life
Cooked meats	3–4 days	2–3 months
Raw meats	1–2 days	3–4 months
Deli sliced meats, opened	3–5 days	1–2 months
Cooked poultry	3–4 days	4–6 months
Raw poultry	1–2 days	9–12 months
Cooked grains	4–5 days	1–2 months
Cooked potato	3–5 days	3–4 months
Cooked fish	2–3 days	2 months
Raw lean fish	1–2 days	6–8 months
Raw fatty fish	1–2 days	2–3 months
Canned fish, opened	3–4 days	2 months
Cooked shrimp	2–3 days	2–3 months
Raw shrimp	1–2 days	3–6 months
Cooked vegetables	3–6 days	2–3 months
Fresh herbs	1 week	2–3 months*
Cooked eggs	3 days	2–3 months
Overnight oats	3–4 days	2–3 months
Stews	3–4 days	2–3 months
Soups	3–4 days	2–3 months
Salad	3–5 days	Not suitable for freezing
Mashed potatoes	3–4 days	2–3 months
Sauces	5 days	2–3 months*
Dips	3–4 days	3–4 months

*The best way to freeze fresh herbs and most sauces is in ice cube trays! Allow sauce to cool to room temperature before pouring into trays. For herbs, pre-cut them and mix with a few drops of water before placing in trays.

GRAINS

Grains expand when cooked and can yield multiple times the dry amount. Bookmark this guide so you know exactly how much to cook and how much liquid you'll be needing.

Grain	Uncooked	Cooked	Liquid
Rice	1 cup (200 g)	3 cups (510 g)	2 cups (475 ml)
Quinoa	1 cup (180 g)	3 cups (555 g)	2 cups (475 ml)
Bulgur	1 cup (150 g)	3 cups (450 g)	2 cups (475 ml)
Pearl barley	1 cup (215 g)	3 cups (645 g)	3 cups (700 ml)
Pearl couscous	1 cup (160 g)	3 cups (540 g)	1¼ cups (300 ml)
Pasta	1 cup (55 g)	2 cups (400 g)	–
Lentils	1 cup (200 g)	3 cups (600 g)	3 cups (700 ml)
Rolled oats	1 cup (90 g)	2 cups (300 g)	2 cups (475 ml)

ANIMAL PROTEINS

As a general rule of thumb, meat and other animal proteins will reduce in weight by about 25 percent when cooked. The amount of juices released when these foods are heated depends on how much fat and moisture the cut contains, as well as the cooking temperature and duration. Higher cooking temperatures

how much money can i expect to spend on groceries?

Because you build your own meals, you also get to set your own budget based on the ingredients you choose to use. You can go with the basics and buy them in bulk as a cost-effective option.

There are a few items that I recommend paying extra attention to in terms of quality because it will make an enormous difference in how your everyday meals taste. For instance, high-quality balsamic vinegar is a true delicacy that you could eat by the spoonful. Protein powder is amazing for quick smoothies, shakes, and as a convenient add-on to meals that aren't rich in protein on their own. If a protein powder tastes chalky, switch to another one. I used to dread it, but it turns out I just hadn't found the right one. With so many options out there, it can just take a little time to find your favorite. Don't enjoy the taste? Consider going with an unflavored one. If you like to use extracts in cooking, always go with a pure option rather than artificial. There's a big difference in taste—imitation extracts tend to have a chemical aftertaste.

add flavor!

Cook grains like rice and quinoa in a mixture of water and low-sodium broth for more savory, flavorful sides. Add finely chopped fresh herbs, such as cilantro or parsley, before serving!

will cause more meat shrinkage. For example, a pound, or 16 ounces (450 g), of raw chicken will yield about 12 ounces (340 g) of cooked chicken. Always take the 25 percent shrinkage into account when planning meals that include meat! Animal proteins are typically 1 to 2 ounces (30 to 60 g) per portion. To make one ounce of cooked meat, poultry, or seafood, the uncooked weight is 1¼ ounces (40 g). For a portion size of 2 ounces (60 g), the raw weight you'll need to plan for will be 2½ ounces (75 g).

uncooked vs. cooked weights

When building your meals, it's essential to understand how the weight of your portions changes before and after cooking.

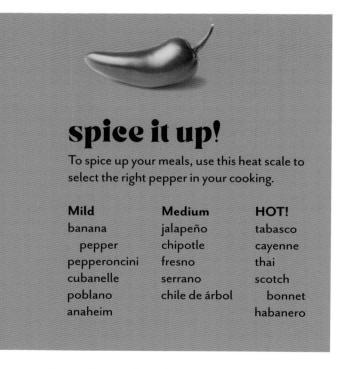

spice it up!

To spice up your meals, use this heat scale to select the right pepper in your cooking.

Mild	Medium	HOT!
banana pepper	jalapeño	tabasco
pepperoncini	chipotle	cayenne
cubanelle	fresno	thai
poblano	serrano	scotch bonnet
anaheim	chile de árbol	habanero

shopping seasonal

I always try to select produce that's in season. In-season produce is perfectly ripe and tastes delicious. It's harvested at its peak, resulting in more flavor and nutrients. Plus, it's more affordable and often farmed locally. Remember, you can also buy produce when it's at its peak and freeze some for later!

PRODUCE STORAGE TIPS

Cool, dark, and dry environment	garlic	pumpkins
	onion	squash
	potatoes	sweet potatoes

Room temperature	fresh basil	tomatoes
	lemons	watermelon
	limes	oranges

Room temperature (transferred to fridge when ripe)	apricots	papaya
	avocados	pears
	kiwis	pineapples
	mangos	plums
	bananas	peaches
	nectarines	plantains

Fridge	apples	cucumber
	asparagus	eggplant
	beets	fresh cilantro
	berries	ginger
	bok choy	lettuce
	broccoli	spinach
	brussels sprouts	kale
	cabbage	mushrooms
	carrots	fresh parsley
	cauliflower	peas
	celery	peppers
	cherries	radishes
	collard greens	scallions
	corn	turnips

WASHING VEGETABLES AND FRUIT

Even organic produce can contain pesticide residue. To clean produce, fill a bowl with water and add a teaspoon of baking soda. Add vegetables or fruit and let soak for a minute or two. Rinse them off with water. Dry them on a clean kitchen towel before storing or eating.

FAQ: HOW CAN I INCORPORATE MORE VEGETABLES INTO MY MEALS IF I DON'T ENJOY SALADS?

Try steaming or roasting your vegetables! Flavor boosters, such as balsamic vinegar, go great with roasted veggies. Here are serving ideas when you need extra inspiration.

VEGETABLE PAIRINGS

Veggie	Steamed	Roasted at 350°F (175°C)	Paired with
Asparagus	5–7 minutes	10–15 minutes	salmon, tuna, casseroles
Bell peppers	6–8 minutes	20–25 minutes	dips, skewers, or stuffed
Broccoli	4–7 minutes	10–15 minutes	steak and potatoes, stir-fry, pasta
Carrots	5–7 minutes	25–35 minutes	dips, pasta sauce, soups
Kale	5 minutes	15–20 minutes	as chips, omelet
Mushrooms	3–5 minutes	15–20 minutes	wraps, pasta sauce, stir-fry
Zucchini	3–5 minutes	15–20 minutes	pasta sauce, zoodles, zucchini boats, grilled with chicken

BACKUP MEAL FIXES

It's a good idea to have a few quick backup choices for the days when you have a jam-packed schedule and can only spare a couple of minutes to put together a tasty meal.

On-the-Go Smoothies

The world of smoothies has something for everyone, and they are so easy to make. To simplify your breakfast or snack, pop smoothie ingredients in a blender and you'll have a delicious meal to go in seconds. Use rolled oats as your starch, nuts or seeds as your healthy fats, and yogurt and protein powder as your sources of protein. Add fruit and water or unsweetened almond milk to mix.

Toss-It-Together Bowls

Bowls equal endless possibilities in practically no time! Use a scoop of rice or quinoa as your base, then top with any proteins and veggies of your choice. Drizzle with your favorite sauce to set the mood of your bowl. For inspiration, check out the recipe for Slow-Cooker Shredded Beef Barbacoa (page 172).

Switch Up the Basics with Sauces

Make two to three sauces or dressings for each week along with a large batch of your favorite proteins and starches from the Meal Builder swap tables to give your meals variety. That way, you always have the option of combining food with a different sauce. You could be having shrimp with Creamy Blender Pesto Sauce (page 189) for lunch and steak with Argentinian-Style Steak with Chimichurri Sauce (page 156) for dinner.

take a journey through food

Variety is the spice of life, and there's never a reason to sacrifice flavor! So, let's get to the good stuff: spices, herbs, and other flavor boosters. One of the best ways to keep your meals exciting and find variety in cooking is by discovering new flavors and trying different cuisines and signature dishes.

Country/region	Flavor boosters	Sauces and add-ons
Argentinian	ají (mild red pepper), basil, cumin, garlic, parsley, oregano, rosemary, smoked paprika, thyme	chimichurri, salsa criolla, salsa tuco
Brazilian	garlic, annatto, chili peppers, cumin, cilantro, onion, paprika, tempero baiano blend, nutmeg	molho apimentado, molho de alho
Chinese	chili peppers, cinnamon, garlic, ginger, scallions, sesame seeds, star anise	soy sauce, oyster sauce, rice wine, rice vinegar, hoisin sauce
Cuban, Puerto Rican, and Dominican	adobo, bay leaf, cilantro, cinnamon, cloves, culantro, cumin, dill, garlic, ginger, lime, nutmeg, oregano, parsley, sweet paprika, thyme	mojo, pique verde, sofrito, wasakaka
French	bay leaves, basil, chives, herbes de Provence, fines herbes, mustard, oregano, paprika, parsley, rosemary, saffron, shallots, tarragon, thyme	Dijon mustard, béchamel sauce, velouté sauce, espagnole sauce, hollandaise sauce
Greek	anise, basil, bay leaf, cloves, dill, fennel, garlic, honey, mint, nutmeg, oregano, parsley, thyme	tzatziki, tahini
Haitian	Creole seasoning, garlic, scallions, parsley, peppers, thyme	sos ti-malice
Indian	cayenne pepper, cloves, garam masala, garlic, fennel, cardamom, turmeric, curry, coriander, nutmeg	masala, coconut curry, curries, chutneys, pakora, samosa
Italian	basil, bay leaf, garlic, lemon, marjoram, oregano, parsley, hot chili flakes, rosemary, sage, thyme	pesto, ragu, marinara, carbonara
Jamaican	garlic, cloves, ginger, jerk seasoning, pimento (allspice), Scotch bonnet peppers, smoked paprika, thyme	mango salsa, BBQ jerk sauce

Japanese	chili peppers, dashi stock, ginger, matcha, mirin, negi, sansho peppers, scallions, sesame, shichimi togarashi, wasabi, yuzu	miso sauce, ponzu sauce, teriyaki, soy sauce
Korean	chili peppers, garlic, ginger, ginseng, dashima (kelp), gochugaru (Korean chili powder), onion, perilla leaves, sesame seeds	Korean BBQ sauce, gochujang, soybean paste sauce
Mexican	chili peppers, cayenne pepper, cilantro, cinnamon, cumin, epazote, garlic, hot pepper flakes, lemon, lime, onion, oregano, saffron, tamarind	pico de gallo, salsa verde, guacamole, adobo sauce
Peruvian	basil, chincho, cilantro, cinnamon, cloves, coriander, cumin, fennel, huacatay (Peruvian black mint), oregano, paico, paprika, marjoram, nutmeg, parsley, thyme, turmeric	ají verde sauce, salsa verde
Scandinavian	basil, chives, cinnamon, cumin, dill, ginger, marjoram, mustard, parsley, tarragon, horseradish, thyme, bay leaf, cardamom, nutmeg, vanilla	cranberry sauce, mustard and dill sauce, remoulade
Spanish	bay leaves, basil, cilantro, garlic, lemon, onion, oregano, paprika, parsley, peppers, rosemary, saffron, thyme	brava, garlic aioli, picada, romesco
Thai	basil, chili peppers, cilantro, coriander, cumin, curry pastes, ginger, lemongrass, lime, mint, tamarind, turmeric	fish sauce, oyster sauce, sweet chili sauce, pad Thai sauce, peanut sauce

seasoning blends

Flavor starts with dynamic spice blends and seasonings. These blends only take minutes to mix together, and they can last from six months to a year stored in an airtight container. Make your blends ahead of time and you'll stay ahead of the game!

Cajun Seasoning
MAKES: ½ CUP (70 G)

A seasoning blend that originates from Louisiana, the home of Cajun cuisine. This popular spicy seasoning goes well with essentially every type of food. Try the One-Pan Cajun Shrimp Penne (page 130) or the Louisiana Pineapple Chicken Foil Packets (page 177)!

3 tablespoons (20 g) smoked paprika
1 tablespoon (5 g) cayenne pepper
2 tablespoons (10 g) garlic powder
1 tablespoon (7 g) onion powder
1 tablespoon (3 g) dried oregano
½ tablespoon (3 g) ground black pepper
½ tablespoon (2 g) dried thyme

Jerk Seasoning Rub
MAKES: ½ CUP (70 G)

Often used as a wet marinade, aromatic Jamaican jerk spice rub adds heat and smoky flavors to chicken, seafood, and pork. Traditionally made with brown sugar, this is a sugar-free version of the seasoning.

1 tablespoon (4 g) dried thyme
1 tablespoon (6 g) ground allspice
2 teaspoons (4 g) garlic powder
1 teaspoon ground cinnamon
1 teaspoon ground cloves
1 teaspoon ground ginger
1 teaspoon ground nutmeg
1 tablespoon (7 g) onion powder
1 teaspoon ground black pepper
1 teaspoon Scotch bonnet chili flakes, or to taste
1 tablespoon (3 g) dried chives

Lemon Pepper
MAKES: ⅔ CUP (40 G)

A staple in all-American seasoning, lemon pepper goes great with chicken. Why buy it in a store when you can make a better than store-bought version at home with just four basic ingredients?

Zest of 5 lemons
3 tablespoons (20 g) ground black pepper
1 tablespoon (7 g) garlic powder
1 tablespoon (7 g) onion powder

Italian Seasoning

MAKES: ⅔ CUP (30 G)

Italian seasoning is the perfect addition to pasta sauces and sprinkled on pizza. It's a flavorful classic to enjoy year-round.

2 tablespoons (10g) dried basil
2 tablespoons (6 g) dried oregano
1 tablespoon (3 g) dried rosemary
2 tablespoons (4 g) dried parsley
1 tablespoon (4 g) dried thyme
1 tablespoon (4 g) red chili flakes, or to taste
1 teaspoon garlic powder

Herbes de Provence

MAKES: 1 CUP (55 G)

Hailing from southeastern France, herbes de Provence is a fragrant spice blend used in French and Mediterranean cooking. It's a great flavor-booster for grilled chicken and fish, roasted veggies, soups and stews, and even salad.

2 tablespoons (6 g) dried rosemary
1 tablespoon (6 g) fennel seed
2 tablespoons (8 g) dried thyme
2 tablespoons (10g) dried basil
2 tablespoons (8 g) dried savory
1 tablespoon (2 g) dried tarragon
1 tablespoon (3 g) dried lavender
1 tablespoon (3 g) dried dill
2 tablespoons (8 g) dried marjoram
2 teaspoons (2 g) dried oregano

everyday flavor boosters

Poultry Blend

MAKES: ¼ CUP (20 G)

1 tablespoon (4 g) dried thyme
½ tablespoon (2 g) dried rosemary
1 tablespoon (2 g) dried sage
1 teaspoon dried marjoram
½ tablespoon (4 g) garlic powder
½ tablespoon (4 g) onion powder
½ teaspoon ground black pepper

Steak Blend

MAKES: ⅓ CUP (35 G)

1 tablespoon (7 g) smoked paprika
1 tablespoon (7 g) onion powder
2 tablespoons (10 g) garlic powder
½ tablespoon (3 g) ground black pepper
2 teaspoons (3 g) dried thyme
2 teaspoons (2 g) dried rosemary

Seafood Blend

MAKES: ⅓ CUP (40 G)

2 tablespoons (7 g) smoked paprika
2 tablespoons (10 g) garlic powder
1 tablespoon (7 g) onion powder
2 teaspoons (3 g) dried thyme
1 teaspoon celery seed
½ teaspoon ground cumin

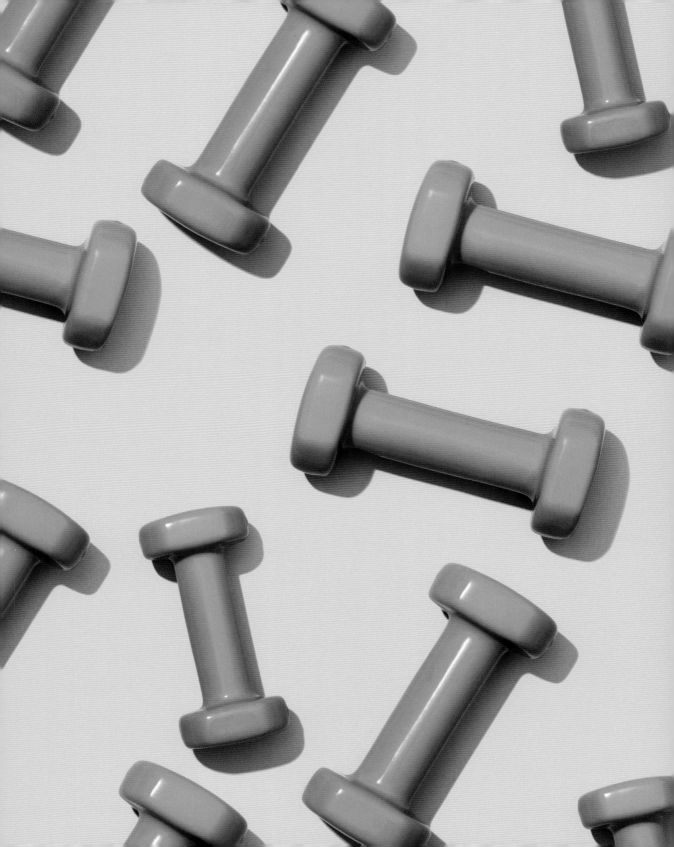

work it out

AS PART OF THE SCULPT PROGRAM, you gain access to an interactive fitness plan that you can keep in your phone, so it goes everywhere with you! To get started, download the app (accessible through thesculptplan.com/book). Within the app, you'll find workouts with detailed descriptions, video demonstrations, and modifications for each exercise. Even better, it allows you to connect with other members who share this fantastic journey with you!

In this chapter, you'll:

- get familiar with the role of exercise in weight loss
- discover the *Sculpt* way of working out
- find ways to work out on a busy schedule
- make a plan B for movement

We know working out has a huge upside for health beyond weight loss—regular exercise has been shown to improve the outcomes of countless diseases and conditions. We also know that it forms part of a balanced lifestyle. The fewer calories you burn, the more likely you are to gain weight, which is why sedentary behavior is so closely linked to excess weight. The more sitting you do in a day, the greater your need for exercise.

When the goal is to lose weight, exercise can:

- help you burn more calories
- reduce body fat
- repair a sluggish metabolism
- increase your lean body mass
- improve your body composition

When incorporated into your lifestyle in the long term, it can:

- help maintain a healthy weight
- increase energy levels
- enhance mental clarity
- improve your mood
- act as a stress reliever
- improve quality of sleep
- make you happier by releasing feel-good hormones
- reduce the risk of chronic conditions and other health problems

does exercise equal weight loss?

It is important to know that any exercise routine is only as good as the eating habits that go along with it. Movement is a key component of a healthy lifestyle, but it hasn't been shown to produce significant weight loss results on its own. This makes sense—we can easily eat hundreds of calories worth of food in just minutes, while it can take hours to burn the same number of calories with exercise (unfair, I know!).

In other words, you can't out-exercise a bad diet. How about vice versa—can you lose weight by adjusting your diet, but without exercising? The short answer is yes. But many studies also suggest that regular physical activity is an important predictor of maintaining weight loss. So, although it's possible to lose weight without working out, there are plenty of reasons to embrace it as part of a balanced, healthy lifestyle.

Being active has an essential role in the *Sculpt* program, because exercise maximizes the number of calories that the body burns throughout the day, allowing you to widen the gap between the calories you consume and the calories you burn. Getting strong benefits your metabolism, too, because muscle burns more calories than fat. The more lean muscle you have, the more calories your body will burn at rest, adding up to the total calories burned in the day.

But the benefits go deeper than physical changes. Committing to caring for your body through planned movement has both physical and mental advantages. And that euphoric feeling you get right after a good workout? On a neurochemical level, exercise stimulates the production of mood-elevating hormones in your brain, which has a unique power to make you feel good, contributing to the stress-relieving benefits of exercise.

easing your way into fitness

If you feel you're not ready to jump headfirst into a full-fledged fitness program, that's okay. We all have different starting points, and what's most important is not the type of exercise you choose but that you stay moving—in any way you enjoy. I used to hate the thought of exercising because I had always forced myself to be active in ways I didn't enjoy. When I stopped doing that, and built my routine around what I actually liked, I fell in love with it.

Consistent lifestyle changes, no matter how small, can make an enormous difference when you keep at it, day after day. So, if you're not ready to claim your spot in the *Sculpt* fitness program just yet, set an achievable goal that you know you can commit to. The important thing is to find something you love! Time-wise, it can be as little as thirty minutes a day doing any physical activity at any intensity, like walking, light jogging, yoga, dancing, biking, swimming, or hiking. Remember, too, that as you lose weight, these activities get easier, more enjoyable, and even—dare I say it—addictive!

working out the sculpt way

With your fitness program through the app, you can work out at home, the gym, or with minimal equipment. The program combines four components: weight training, sculpting sessions, metabolic training, and cardio. There are six weekly options available. You don't have to complete all of them, but I encourage you to take advantage of your free months and try to fit in as many sessions per week as your schedule allows.

While it's perfectly fine to start with using your bodyweight only, if you are looking to build your home workout space, there are a few items I highly recommend investing in to get the most out of your program: a yoga mat, weights (ideally one lighter set and one heavier set), loop resistance bands, and a resistance tube with handles.

SCULPTING SESSIONS

My attitude toward working out changed when I realized I didn't need gym machines for a training session to be effective. Sculpting sessions are a great example of that. They include targeted workouts for the upper and lower body that will make you feel the burn with resistance band work and exercises that focus on bodyweight. If you're experienced with training, you can modify the moves to be more challenging by adding in a pair of ankle weights. But don't underestimate the power of resistance bands alone—they make all the difference in your workouts.

Loop bands, also known as mini bands, or booty bands, are fantastic for waking up your leg and glute muscles before a workout, essentially telling them to get ready to work! You can use them to add extra resistance to any exercise without having to increase weight. They come in latex and fabric—either one does the job. If you exercise mainly at home, I highly recommend getting a resistance tube with handles. It's a versatile tool for toning arms and back that provides the security of a sturdy grip, and you can use it to replace many weighted upper body exercises that you'd typically need gym equipment for.

Equipment essentials: loop bands, resistance tube with handles, yoga mat

Optional: ankle weights

METABOLIC TRAINING

We've talked a lot about boosting your metabolism throughout this book, and metabolic training plays a key role in just that. It consists of quick workout sessions designed especially for those days when you're very short on time, allowing you to maximize the time you spend exercising by multiplying the calories you burn.

Metabolic training pairs weight training and cardio through intense exercise intervals, training the body to burn more calories at rest post-workout. These sessions are much more concentrated than traditional cardio or weight training sessions, but

they allow you to build lean muscle and shed excess fat even more efficiently.

Equipment essentials: a set of weights

Optional: kettlebell, barbell

WEIGHT TRAINING

Don't let the name scare you! As you may have guessed, weight training requires the body to move against an opposing force, whether it's dumbbells, a kettlebell, a barbell, or any other element you choose to use as weight. Building lean muscle through resistance training helps boost your metabolism, and having toned muscles can reduce the appearance of loose, saggy skin. Paired with cardio and healthy eating habits, it can also reduce the appearance of cellulite. Like metabolic training, lifting weights can increase your basal metabolic rate and your body continues to burn more calories throughout the day, even when you're not training. Talk about maximizing your time!

Equipment essentials: a set of weights

Optional: kettlebell, barbell

choosing your weights

When selecting weights, ask yourself two questions: Does this weight feel challenging, and am I still able to perform high quality repetitions with good form? It's important to choose a weight that challenges you but one that still allows you to complete each repetition with controlled movement.

If you train at a gym, you can always ask for guidance from a staff member or personal trainer. If you work out at home, aim to get two sets of dumbbells as you build your workout space: lighter weights for the upper body, and heavier weights for the lower body. You can also consider getting just one set of adjustable dumbbells. If you don't have access to weights, get creative and use anything you can find—even water bottles or food cans will do!

Will Weight Training Make Me Look Bulky?

No, incorporating weight training into your fitness regime with the *Sculpt* fitness plan won't make you bulk up! In fact, weight training tightens, tones, and burns fat efficiently. There is a common misconception that lifting weights will make the female body look "bulky," causing many women to stick exclusively to cardio. However, in recent years, we've seen more women picking up weights, as that myth fades away. The reality is that it would take eating significantly more calories than you burn—also known as a caloric surplus—and a whole lot of time in the gym to build that kind of muscle. Even then, it would be a challenging task!

HIIT CARDIO

HIIT stands for high-intensity interval training, which elevates your heart rate quickly to burn more calories in less time. HIIT sessions are similar to metabolic training—intense workouts that only last twenty to thirty minutes on average, making them ideal for those days when you're pressed for time. Like metabolic training, HIIT increases the body's need for oxygen during the workout, causing an afterburn effect called *excess post-exercise oxygen consumption* (EPOC), which is why this intense style burns calories so efficiently.

Optional: jump rope

LISS CARDIO

Unlike HIIT, low-intensity steady-state cardio (LISS) is performed at a consistent pace, around 50 to 60 percent of your maximum heart rate. It includes low-impact activities like brisk walking, taking a dance class, swimming, biking, or light jogging.

If you can maintain a casual conversation throughout your LISS session without struggling to catch your breath, you're doing it right! If you're getting out of breath, slow down a bit until you're at a comfortable, steady speed. Because this exercise is gentle on the knees and joints, it's a great option for those who have more weight to lose. LISS sessions typically last anywhere from thirty to sixty minutes.

DON'T FORGET TO STRETCH!

When you access your workouts on the app, you'll see warm-up sessions to prep muscles for exercise and cool-downs to finish off strong. When things get busy, it's easy to forget about stretching and warming up. But here's the thing: Prioritizing mobility can make or break your workout, literally. Stretching reduces the possibility of injury, improves posture, form, and flexibility, and boosts joint health. And as a bonus, it increases the blood flow to your muscles, helping you feel more relaxed and less stressed after exercising.

TAKE A DAY OFF

As important as movement is, taking time to recover is equally necessary. Rest days give your muscles,

bonus tracker (optional)

Keeping a workout tracker can be a huge help! Use the exercise tracker on the next page to log the type of workout, start and finish time, duration, along with the number of sets, reps, and weights used to challenge yourself with every new workout.

exercise tracker and planner

DATE: START TIME: FINISH TIME:

TYPE OF WORKOUT: FOCUS: DURATION:

Exercise	Set #1 reps/weight	Set #2 reps/weight	Set #3 reps/weight	Set #4 reps/weight

DATE: START TIME: FINISH TIME:

TYPE OF MOVEMENT: FOCUS: DURATION:

Exercise	Set #1 reps/weight	Set #2 reps/weight	Set #3 reps/weight	Set #4 reps/weight

S	M	T	W	T	F	S	Workout
○	○	○	○	○	○	○	Sculpting session
○	○	○	○	○	○	○	Weight training
○	○	○	○	○	○	○	Metabolic training
○	○	○	○	○	○	○	LISS cardio
○	○	○	○	○	○	○	HIIT cardio
○	○	○	○	○	○	○	Brisk walk
○	○	○	○	○	○	○	Other:

nerves, bones, and connective tissues time to recover and rebuild. Excessive exercise without rest days in between can lead to injuries, fatigue, hormonal alterations, a lowered immune system, and worse sleep.

You should have at least one day of full rest per week and lower the intensity of your workouts on two to three days out of the week. Feeling overwhelmed? Remember that it's okay to start slow. Your body is undergoing amazing changes—you've got this!

FITTING IN YOUR WORKOUTS

When your schedule gets hectic, you may be tempted to knock workouts off your calendar. To simply tell you to prioritize exercising would be hypocritical of me because I used to be the first person to cancel a session! Something would always get in the way of me and my workouts—that's until I did something about it.

my excuse-proof list for fitting in a workout (even when life gets wild)

1   **BREAK UP YOUR SESSIONS.** Did you know that you don't actually need to exercise for thirty or forty-five consecutive minutes to benefit from it? You can split the time into ten- or fifteen-minute exercise blocks on days that you're running low on time and complete them when it best works for you.

2   **TREAT YOUR WORKOUT AS AN APPOINTMENT.** As simple as it may sound, book time for your workouts in your calendar. Treating them with the same level of priority that you'd give any other appointment makes it more likely for you to follow through. To help organize your time properly, fill out a weekly calendar of planned movement on the previous

page. Doing this will also help you track how much activity you're getting each week!

3   **SET UP YOUR HOME WORKOUT SPACE.** Create your own fitness space at home! Even if it's just a little corner, have your yoga mat, resistance bands, and other home workout gear set up in a designated spot. However big or small the size of your space, having an area dedicated solely to exercising at home makes it a lot easier to fit in your workouts even on the busiest days.

4   **DON'T OVERCOMPLICATE IT.** Find an activity you actually enjoy doing! The more you look forward to exercising, the more probable it is that you'll do it. If your working hours are irregular, don't sign up for a fitness class that starts at the same time each week. Instead, aim for activities that can be easily slotted into your day, like getting steps in during lunch, parking your car some blocks away from the supermarket to add an extra walk, or getting off the train or bus a stop or two early.

5   **GET A WORKOUT BUDDY.** Having another person to stay active with helps you stay accountable with daily movement, making you less likely to ditch your workouts. Together, commit to working out a certain number of times a week, by meeting up or just checking in on each other on days when your schedules don't match. Having a virtual workout buddy works just as well! When you know someone else is counting on you and that person will notice if you didn't show up, you'll hold yourself accountable, too.

6   **SET UP THE NIGHT BEFORE.** Planning ahead goes a long way! When you're in a hurry, the last thing you want is to be hunting around for your workout clothes. Keep all your fitness outfits in the same area of your wardrobe so you can find them quickly when it's time to go. If you exercise in the morning, set your workout clothes by the bed the

night before, or pack your gym bag in advance and have it ready to go by the front door.

7 **REWARD YOURSELF.** Rewards can make sticking to your workouts so much more motivating and fun! Whether it's gifting yourself a cute new workout top, home fitness gear, or getting a massage for accomplishing goals you've set for yourself, positive reinforcements have a way of making new habits stick. And if you're not looking to splurge, it doesn't have to be costly. A relaxing bubble bath, going to the movies, creating a new workout playlist, or taking the time to read a new book can serve as a motivation boost to keep going!

exercise and stress

Most of us live under constant stress. Our bodies release a stress hormone called cortisol when we feel pressure from a person, a situation, or an environment. Chronic stress and high cortisol levels are linked to weight gain and excess weight, along with high blood pressure, heart disease, anxiety, and depression.

But what explains the connection between stress and weight? Cortisol is in charge of regulating your metabolism, blood sugar levels, inflammation, and other immune responses, which is why stress actually has the power to hinder your weight loss results.

And the stress-relieving benefits of exercise aren't talked about nearly enough. There's a simple scientific explanation for how amazing and stress-free you feel after pushing your limits: Exercise can actually help your brain deal with stress more productively. Because it's such an important part of losing weight, we will talk about stress management in more detail in chapter 9!

walk your way into fitness

If you haven't been active in a while, going from sedentary to sporty overnight can feel like a daunting challenge. But I have good news for you—exercise doesn't have to be ultra-intense to produce amazing results, and you certainly don't have to start from an advanced level. If you are struggling with completing your workouts, brisk walking can be your plan B to start with. Walking is one of the most beneficial forms of low-impact exercise, it requires no special gear or prior fitness experience, and you can literally do it anywhere and anytime. Just put on your sneakers and go!

Even if you're completing your workouts in the app, taking a walk on an active rest day, or choosing it as your LISS cardio option, walking has great physical and mental benefits. Most smartphones today come with a built-in step tracker—make a habit of tracking your daily steps. Remember that we all begin our journey from a different point, and if you need to start from ten minutes a day, it still very much counts! Start where you feel comfortable, and from there, add to your walks each day.

STEP UP YOUR GAME

Are you up for a challenge? Once you've created a routine out of daily walks, gradually increase their length and intensity. Start with a goal of 3,000 steps a day for a week, then add an extra 1,000 steps each following week until you reach 10,000 daily steps!

To dial up the intensity, try intervals alternating between a fast pace and a steady pace. Walk as fast as you can for thirty seconds. Slow down to a steady pace for thirty seconds. Then, work your way up to longer fast-paced times while keeping the slow-paced times the same.

thrive!

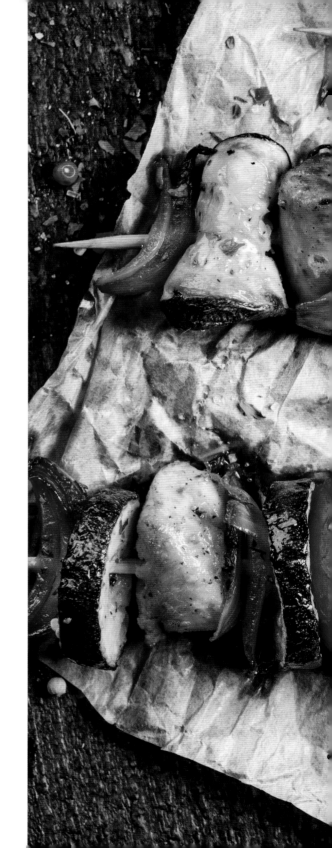

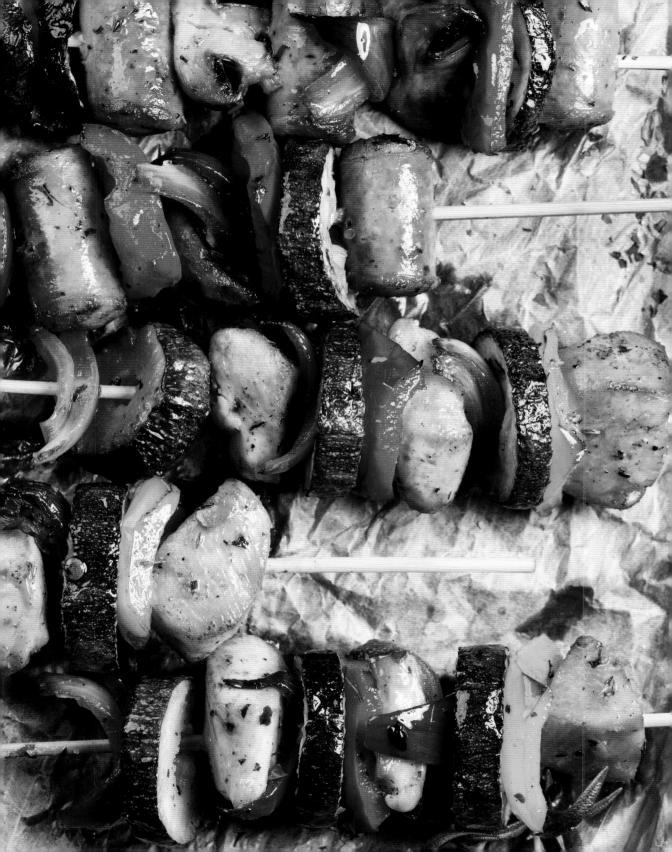

keeping your balance (no matter what)

IT'S SAFE TO SAY THAT there's much more to weight loss than just eating less and moving more. By focusing on calories alone, we'd be unlikely to maintain results in the long run—simply because as human beings, we don't only run on fuel. Sure, your energy balance ultimately determines the way your body composition changes, but your quality of sleep, ways of managing stress, and how you care for your body all fall under the same category of factors that contribute to your weight and overall health.

In this chapter, we will dive into the lifestyle pillars that can affect both weight loss and maintenance, backed by science. Some of the topics we will talk about include:

- creating a bedtime routine for better sleep
- strategies for stress management
- enjoying occasional indulgences
- getting back on track after a break

The ultimate purpose of the program is to give you a complete set of tools to help you thrive as you are losing weight and for the rest of your life! But sometimes, life throws a curveball. When things go awry, you can rely on this chapter to support you.

creating a better bedtime routine

So far, you've been taking care of yourself by fueling your body with nourishing foods and finding joy in movement, which are two cornerstones of optimal health. And I bet you can guess the third: good sleep. We all know that a consistent good night's sleep is a key part of a healthy lifestyle, though we so often neglect it. According to the CDC, one in three American adults do not get enough sleep. Good sleep isn't just about the hours you clock, either. It's about falling asleep and sleeping restfully through the night.

If you're wondering what sleep has to do with your weight loss journey, the two are actually quite

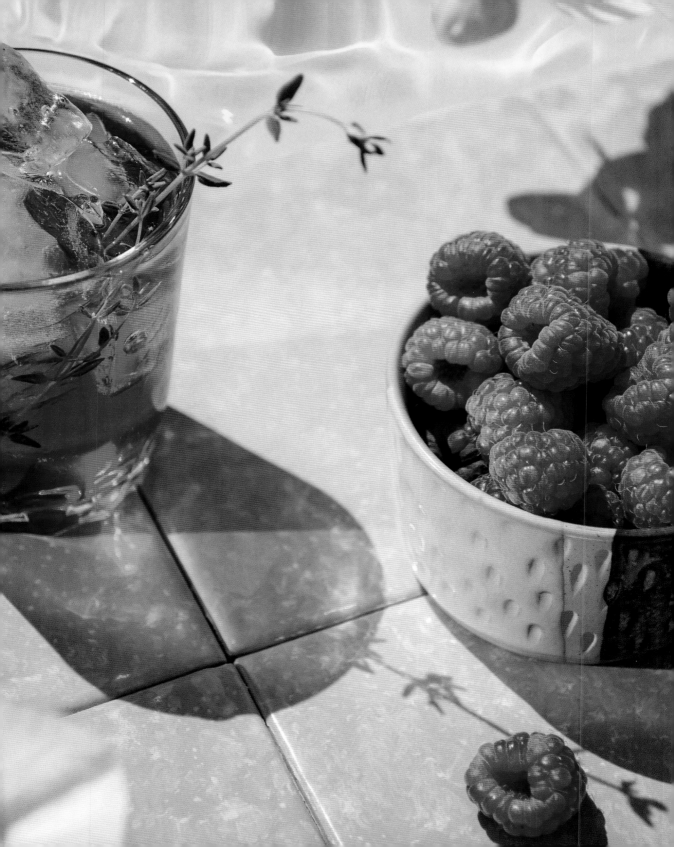

connected. Many studies have shown an association between sleep deprivation and weight gain. And it doesn't take long—poor sleep can affect your weight loss results in as little as two weeks. One study even reported that missing a few hours of sleep for just one night can push you to eat over 550 more calories the next day! In theory, that could lead to a pound of weight gain in just a week.

I'm sure you've noticed that you tend to feel hungrier and have more cravings for high-calorie foods after spending the night tossing and turning, often wanting to eat more and exercise less. And it's not just you! Science says there's a reason for it: Lack of sleep can disrupt the hormonal regulation of your appetite. If you are continuously getting too little sleep, you're less likely to make positive decisions when it comes to eating and staying active.

So, what's the secret to quality sleep even when your days are long and hectic? While you can't add more hours to the day, you do have the power to make those hours count and work to your advantage. By intentionally creating productive routines and removing the roadblocks that are preventing you from getting a solid seven to nine hours of sleep a night, making time for the things you want to achieve while getting good rest becomes less of a hassle. Give these sleep-inducing strategies a try!

REVAMP YOUR BEDTIME ROUTINE FOR BETTER SLEEP

Unplug Yourself from Devices

It's easy to lose track of evening hours to social media scrolling and late-night email checking. For better sleep, go fully technology-free by putting away your phone, laptop, TV, or tablet thirty to sixty minutes before bedtime. The blue light from electronics can mess with sleep cues by disrupting melatonin-regulating sleep hormones. Plus, receiving high volumes of information late at night makes it hard to switch off your brain and enter a peaceful rest mode. Toss the remote and grab your bullet journal (page 43) instead! Even a few minutes of journaling can help calm anxious thoughts and get you more relaxed for bed.

Watch Your Caffeine

While caffeine can be a good pick-me-up during the day, it's no secret that it can disrupt your sleep. Your Meal Builder doesn't incorporate any foods or beverages with significant amounts of caffeine, but if you consume drinks like coffee, avoid them for at least four to six hours before bedtime. If you're sensitive to caffeine, consider cutting it out as early as noon or eliminating it completely.

Relax Your Mind

Do something that you actually enjoy before bed, even if it's for just fifteen or twenty minutes! This doesn't have to involve drinking tea or doing yoga—although it certainly can! It's any moment of relaxation that you take the time to create for yourself, like taking a hot bath, reading a book, cuddling with your pet, or trying a quick meditation (next page). Meditating at night is fantastic if you have trouble falling asleep—it naturally increases the production of the sleep hormone melatonin.

Set a Bedtime (and Keep It!)

Bedtime isn't just for kids! When you plan what time you'll be going to bed, you'll notice how much easier structuring the rest of the evening becomes. Having a regular bedtime puts you in charge of resetting your sleep routine, improving sleep quality, and training your body to sleep more restfully. And if you can't fall asleep right away, go back to the last tip and try doing something relaxing before attempting it again.

tools to managing stress

In addition to sleep, stress is another determining factor that regulates weight. When left unchecked, it can negatively contribute to nearly every known health problem. Stress drives our eating behaviors, and it can even control the rate at which we lose or gain weight. Just like a night of bad sleep, studies show that higher stress levels often lead to craving sugary or greasy foods, making it more difficult to stick to healthy habits. Food can feel like an easy outlet for seeking comfort when life gets hard, but as we know from chapter 3, this can turn into a counterproductive loop of emotional eating that undermines our goals.

Unfortunately, we all have some level of stress in our lives. Often there isn't much we can do about the length of our to-do lists, but we can find ways to cope that don't involve soothing stress with food. Here's how to break the cycle and feel more in control when faced with difficult situations.

Be in the Moment

Sometimes all you need is a breather. And I mean that literally: Behavioral scientists have found that a technique as simple as taking deep breaths in a stressful situation can immediately lower your anxiety levels. Meditation and mindfulness can help you rechannel stress, control thoughts from bouncing around, and look at reality from a more grounded, objective, and manageable place. Contrary to popular belief, meditation is not about eliminating your thoughts. It's about being aware of them and letting them pass without judgment, connecting to the present moment. By helping you get to a place of self-awareness, it can enable you to make better choices in a tough spot. Are you ready to give it a shot?

Five-Minute Meditations

You'll only need five minutes for these simple meditation exercises. They can instantly help you feel calmer and more centered by lowering the stress hormone cortisol. You can do them anywhere, anytime! If right now is not a good time, bookmark this page and save it for later to apply when you're feeling defeated, have trouble falling asleep, or just need to collect your thoughts.

To begin, select one of the challenges below and set a timer for five minutes. Find a comfortable place to sit, preferably with your eyes closed. Concentrate on breathing: Shallow breaths tell the body you're in fight-or-flight mode, while deep breaths that come from the belly are comforting by relaying to the mind that all is well. That's what makes something as easy as deep breathing essential for managing nerve-racking situations.

Keep in mind that the goal of these exercises is to observe your thoughts, not to hang onto them or stop them.

Breathing Challenge

Inhale deeply from the belly to the count of 1, 2, 3, 4. Then, exhale to the count of 4, 3, 2, 1. Place a hand on your stomach and feel it expand as you inhale. Repeat until the timer goes off.

Counting Your Breaths Challenge

Count every deep breath you take in and exhale from the belly. Place a hand on your stomach and feel it expand as you inhale. Keep counting, and if you lose count, start over until your timer goes off.

Mind Observing Challenge

Taking deep breaths, expand your lungs on each inhale and lower on the exhale. Concentrate on breathing from the belly. Place a hand on your stomach and feel it expand as you inhale. Connect with your thoughts and physical sensations. As you do this, your mind may wander. If it does, gently bring it back. Notice what you hear, see, smell, and feel. Continue observing your environment until your timer goes off.

Body Observing Challenge

Taking deep breaths, expand your lungs on each inhale and lower them on the exhale. Concentrate on breathing from the belly. Place a hand on your stomach and feel it expand when you inhale. Focus your attention on different parts of your body, in order. Notice your toes, heels, ankles, legs and knees, hips and stomach, chest, back, shoulders, arms, and hands, and finally your head and face. Then, start from your face and head, working your way down to your toes. Repeat until the timer goes off.

Mindfulness goes beyond meditation. In the last chapter, we touched on the role of movement and exercise in relieving stress through endorphins, the feel-good hormones. But even before getting to that post-workout euphoria, the simple act of taking the time to exercise can distract your mind from worries, placing the focus from your stressors to moving your body. When you incorporate mindful movement consistently each day, you'll notice your tension slowly being replaced with positive energy and sharpened focus.

Similarly, mindfulness can be applied to eating. Think about the last thing you ate. What did it look like? How did it smell? What did it taste like when you took a bite? How did you feel after eating? When we're eating on autopilot, we rarely stop to think about food as we scroll our phones or watch TV. The problem with multitasking while you eat is that it can get difficult to identify when you're full. Being present at mealtimes increases your awareness so you can eat with more pleasure and feel more in control of your eating.

SWITCH UP YOUR SKINCARE

Glowing skin is a big bonus of cultivating healthier habits. As the largest organ of the body, your skin will thank you for matching it with a care regimen to support your lifestyle: lock in moisture, prevent breakouts, and purify your pores after intense workout sessions. No matter what your skin type is, cleansing, exfoliating, and hydrating each have a special role in keeping your complexion bright and clear. Give your skin some extra TLC with the at-home beauty treatments on the next page. They use ingredients you probably have sitting in your pantry right now!

TAKING A BREAK

Unexpected events can happen and throw you off your regular habits. But breaks aren't always bad or unwelcome. As an essential part of life, I want you to be able to go out to a restaurant and celebrate a birthday or take a vacation without feeling guilty. Whether you have a sweet tooth or a soft spot for salty things, enjoying those fun foods now and then is crucial for establishing a lasting positive relationship with food. No need to kiss your goals goodbye—an occasional meal won't make or break your overall journey, no matter what phase of the program you are in.

Allowing yourself to enjoy the foods you love is essential to being able to live a balanced, healthy lifestyle and getting results that last. In fact, some of the most frequently asked questions we get at *Sculpt* are precisely about moments of indulging. Because I've been there myself, I understand why it can raise concern—you've been dedicating all this time to living a healthier life and learning how different foods benefit your progress, so temporarily loosening the grip you've had over your eating can almost feel like undoing all the hard work.

Here's how to enjoy celebrations without feeling like you're going off the rails:

BE MINDFUL OF WHEN YOU FEEL FULL. These events may be centered around food, but indulging doesn't mean you have to eat until you feel totally stuffed. Overeating won't make special moments any more enjoyable or add extra value to them.

KEEP YOUR REGULAR MEAL SCHEDULE. Don't skip any meals leading up to dining out. On many occasions, overeating happens because of irregular mealtimes and unstructured eating during the rest of the day.

BE PRESENT. Concentrate on making memories with the people around you! Whatever you are eating, enjoy every bite, and you're bound to have a much better time. Plus, research shows that when we're present in the moment, we're also more connected to our internal hunger cues.

RETURN TO YOUR REGULAR ROUTINE AFTER. It's time to put the meal behind you and focus on healthier, energizing options for your upcoming meals. Getting back to routine right away ensures that indulging doesn't become a self-sabotaging habit, but rather a fun thing that can be repeated again, fully guilt-free!

eating out

I often hear from people who eat out frequently because of work and struggle with staying on track with healthy eating. I touched on this briefly in chapter 6, where I shared a model to follow when you get to build your own plate. But that's not always possible, especially when you have limited options to choose from. Restaurant portions are often oversized, and it can get challenging to monitor the ingredients and means of preparation when eating out.

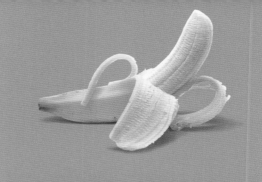

avocado banana hydration bomb

¼ ripe avocado
½ ripe banana
2 tablespoons (25 g) plain yogurt
1 teaspoon honey

Slice the avocado and banana. Mix all the ingredients in a blender. Blend until smooth. Apply evenly on the face. Leave on for 10 to 15 minutes before rinsing with lukewarm water.

coconut coffee body polish

½ cup (40 g) ground coffee beans
¼ cup (70 g) sea salt
2 tablespoons (30 g) coconut oil
½ teaspoon vanilla extract, optional

Mix all the ingredients in a small bowl. If you want the body polish to leave a vanilla scent, add in vanilla extract. Once your skin is wet in the shower, scrub your body with the paste in circular motions for a few minutes before rinsing.

By making a couple of adjustments and preparing a little in advance, these simple tips allow you to keep your thoughts on the actual lunch, and less on what's going on your plate when the intention isn't to indulge.

Eat a Snack Before

Take advantage of switching your meals around your lunch. Have your AM or PM snack from the Meal Builder beforehand, so you won't arrive on an empty stomach. This way, you can order a lighter dish, like an appetizer, if the restaurant doesn't have ideal menu options to choose from. Plus, if you arrive hungry, you're more likely to eat more than your Meal Builder portions' worth.

Make Healthier Swaps

Healthy swaps can be as simple as choosing steamed vegetables over french fries or choosing red pasta sauce instead of white. Typically, white sauces are made with heavy cream, making them dense in saturated fat. Red sauces are tomato-based and a less calorie-dense alternative. Small changes can make a big difference! To save time deciding, check the restaurant's menu and decide what you're going to order ahead of time. Exploring your options before getting to the restaurant makes it easier to find a dish that works best for you.

Make Produce the Star

One sure way to make your restaurant meal more filling is by choosing nutrient-dense non-starchy veggies on the side. Think steamed broccoli, sautéed spinach, roasted eggplant, or a salad as a side for protein-rich foods like grilled chicken or blackened seafood. For dessert, many restaurants can offer a bowl of fruit even if it's not on the list. Plus, fiber-packed fruit will help you feel full longer, but it can also keep you regular, lower your cholesterol, and control blood sugar levels.

Use On-the-Go Portioning

Using a kitchen scale and measuring cups makes portioning your meals a breeze at home, but figuring out portion sizes gets trickier when eating out. Using your hand as a portion guide can serve as an estimation hack when you're looking to follow your Meal Builder as closely as possible.

Cupped Hand = ½ cup
Example: a serving of cooked rice

Clenched Fist = 1 cup
Example: a serving of mixed greens

Palm = 3–4 ounces (85–115 g) meat
Example: a serving of grilled chicken

Thumb = 1 tablespoon
Example: a serving of dressing

Fingertip = 1 teaspoon
Example: a serving of olive oil

restarting the program

Like most things in life, losing weight isn't a straight line. I get it, life happens. Sometimes, a break may last a day or two because of an exceptionally busy work schedule. Other times, maybe there was a big change in your personal life and you had to take a longer break. It's not always easy to jump right back into healthy habits, so I want you to have the tools to find your way back to routine if you ever need to.

Setbacks aren't fun, but one thing is for sure: We all go through them. What matters is what you do about getting back on your feet. Instead of focusing on feeling frustrated or disappointed, think about how far you've come. You've done this before, and you can absolutely do it again!

Revisit Your Reason

Reconnecting with why you started and how you felt before embarking on this journey will be the sustaining force behind the positive changes you've made. Do you still recall your ultimate reason for wanting to do this? I think about how miserable I used to feel every day, both physically and mentally, and how I didn't feel confident being around people or wearing certain clothes. My reason is that I never want to feel like that again!

Reminding yourself of your reason helps keep you going when you're not feeling as motivated, as the big picture can sometimes get buried beneath everything else you've got going on. Because motivation comes in waves, keep visualizing the version of you that you want to become as you continue to push toward your goals.

Kick Things Off with Tracking

The longer your break has been, the more overwhelming the thought of returning to routine can feel. Nutrition is the foundation of a healthy lifestyle, and other pieces of the puzzle tend to fall into place once your eating habits are back in check. But for many people, nutrition is often the most difficult part. During your first week following a break, try logging every meal. While tracking isn't a must in this program, it can be a helpful tool in getting back into the swing of things.

Plan, Plan, Plan!

As we saw in chapter 7, planning your meals ahead of time is key for successful grocery shopping and having healthy meals on hand. With make-ahead meals, it's easier to eat consistently. The same goes for movement—schedule your workouts ahead of time.

Don't Overdo It

Avoid setting yourself up for failure by setting unrealistic goals. Don't try to compensate for a missed workout by working out twice as long the next day or restricting your calories to make up for a larger dinner. Instead of beating yourself up, think of that meal as extra energy that you can use for your next workout.

Set Goals in Steps

After a break, start with smaller goals. Each day, build upon what you accomplished the day before by attaching a new goal to it. For example, if your goal is to start exercising again, start with a short walk on the first day. On the second day, make it your goal to walk for fifteen minutes after lunch. On the third day, aim to take 3,000 steps on your post-lunch walk. On the fourth day, pick up the pace or add ankle weights. Before you know it, you'll be back to your full workout regimen!

What I'd love for you to take away from this chapter is that living the *Sculpt* lifestyle is a journey, rather than a destination. I want to stick to it, not only to maintain my happy weight, but to continue experiencing that magical feeling that comes from nourishing and taking care of my body. I hope that you choose to make yourself your number one priority—before and after reaching your goals.

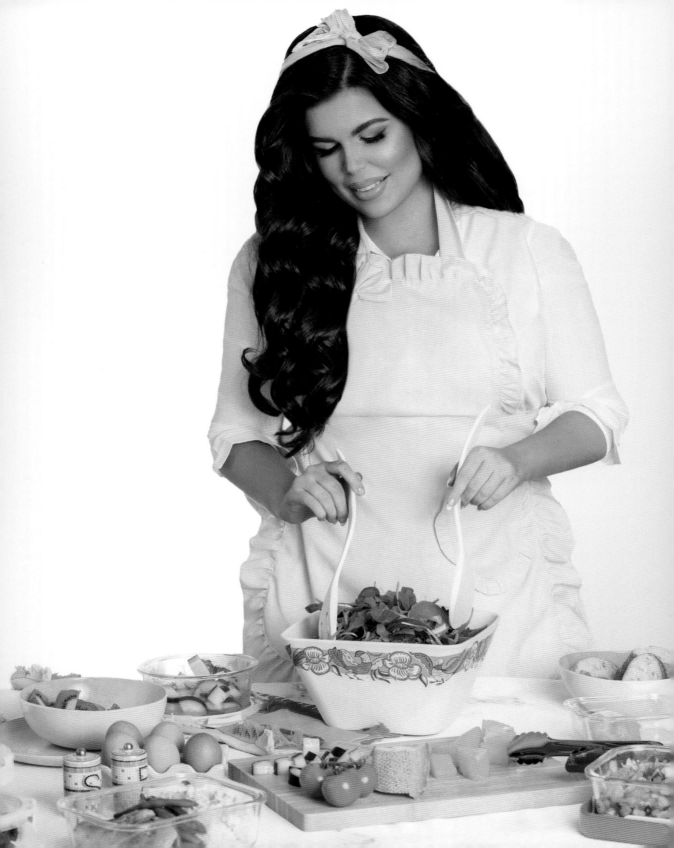

sculpted for life

CONGRATULATIONS, YOU'VE MADE IT to the final chapter! You're here either because you lost the weight you set out to lose in the beginning of the program, or you want to know how your lifestyle will change once you make the shift from weight loss into maintenance mode. We'll kick things off by reflecting on how far you've come.

There's only one person to thank for making it here: yourself! You did it by learning a new way of eating that benefits you. You've made peace with food through breaking down old habits and consistently building new ones. You've pushed yourself, accomplishing goal after goal. Getting here is no small feat! I bet you feel amazing—in fact, the polar opposite of how you felt when you started the program.

This journey has revealed more to you about your potential, hasn't it? By the time I switched to maintenance, I felt as if my life had been divided into two; life before and after the program, all because of how big of an improvement it made in every aspect of my life, well beyond losing weight. And it shows inside and out: your body, mindset, mood, productivity, and energy levels, as well as glowier skin, shinier hair, and stronger nails. Just think about how much you have achieved since you started putting yourself first!

shifting from weight loss to maintenance

Right now, you might be feeling a little nervous. *What if I go back to my old habits now that I've lost the weight?* Not to worry. I wasn't kidding when I told you that our journey together wouldn't end when you reached your happy weight!

Losing weight was just the beginning of your new lifestyle. Now, we focus on maintaining the results that you've earned. You've already done the hardest part: building new healthy habits from scratch. From here on out, as we get into the maintenance mindset, we will reinforce those habits and build on them to make them even stronger.

In this final phase, the goal is no longer to lose weight. We are going to slowly increase your daily food intake each week until you feel in control and comfortable with a more flexible approach to eating. Because everyone's sweet spot for weight maintenance is different, I'm including a set of tools that will help you find yours.

WHY YOU NEED A MAINTENANCE PLAN

You and I both know from personal experience that keeping weight off can be challenging. So do most people who have lost weight—about 95 percent of them, to be exact. If you think about your own journey, the more weight loss attempts you had under your belt, the harder it got to lose weight and maintain the results, didn't it? When I think about my own struggles with dieting through most of my adult life, as discouraging as the numbers are, they make total sense. So, what now? How can we ensure that you will be among the 5 percent of people who do maintain weight loss in the long run? Let's get into it.

You've witnessed the changes in your body with your own eyes as you've lost weight. But here's where you need to focus your attention: Your body has changed on the inside, too. These internal changes are crucial for understanding weight maintenance and taking them into consideration is what makes the difference.

Remember how we said in chapter 5 that during weight loss, your body burns more calories than the calories you ingest through food, and that results in a process called metabolic adaptation? Simply put, the lighter you are, the fewer calories your body needs to burn to function—as your weight decreases, your energy expenditure will need to follow that same path. Now, your body's energy needs have become less than they were at your starting point, as it now has less body mass to maintain. That's the body's natural way of saying that it needs a smaller supply of calories than it did when you were at your starting weight. Because the degree of metabolic adaptation varies from person to person, every person's maintenance level is unique.

When someone who has successfully lost weight returns to poor eating habits despite the metabolic adaptation process that has taken place, they are essentially putting their metabolism through a state of shock and overloading it to the point where the body reacts by hoarding more body fat, followed by rapid weight gain. To avoid this scenario, it's important to give your metabolism a chance to adapt to the changes gradually.

meet the maintenance plan

When I started my formal education in nutrition, two things were clear to me from day one. I would specialize in weight management, and within that field, my focus area would be weight maintenance. I wanted to understand what made the percentage of weight regain so outrageously high among people who had lost weight, and what solutions were needed for the results of weight loss to stick for good.

Alongside my team of nutrition professionals, I regularly participate in national and international conferences to keep up with the latest advances in research around weight management, always with the objective of translating science into practice and real-life solutions. So, you don't need a nutrition degree to figure out any part of the process. We've done the work for you!

The maintenance phase is built around the latest science in nutrition and behavioral change. And like the earlier phases of the program, it's made to fit your life and favorite foods. The strategy is simple: You will add familiar portions of starch, protein, fat, and fruit to your current meals, while documenting your body's response to the changes each week until reaching your maintenance level.

On the first week, you'll start by adding one of these add-ons to the Group 1 Meal Builder daily meals:

½ portion of starch

1 portion of protein

1 portion of fat

1 portion of fruit

Flip to pages 64–67 to refresh your memory on the food swap options! You can choose to pick a different add-on each day or stick to the same one based on what you feel like eating. It doesn't have to be the same food every day! You'll have one add-on on the first week of maintenance.

At the end of the week, weigh yourself and fill out the table below (or on a copy of this page). Simply fill in your week number, current total of add-ons, and mark an X in the box that best describes your weight status.

You'll then adjust your meals for the following week using these steps:

IF YOU'VE LOST 2 POUNDS (1 KG) OR MORE (blue level), incorporate 2 add-ons instead of 1 to your current meals this week. Because we're not looking to lose more weight, blue signals that there is room for 2 add-ons in the coming week.

IF YOUR WEIGHT HAS REMAINED STABLE (green level), or you've gained less than 2 pounds (1 kg), continue adding 1 additional food item from the list. The 2-pound (1 kg) mark considers natural weight fluctuations and indicates that there is room for more add-ons this week.

IF YOU'VE GAINED 2 POUNDS (1 KG) OR MORE (orange level), remove 1 add-on from your weekly meals (if you're on week 1, simply return to the Meal Builder for Group 1 for the week). Orange signals that the previous week's add-on has exceeded your maintenance level and your meals need this adjustment.

Just like in the previous phase, I recommend skipping weigh-ins on the days leading up to and during your period, as you may experience temporary weight fluctuations. Instead, continue logging your weight the following week.

Repeat this self-assessment at the end of each week. Continue adjusting your weekly number of add-ons according to the instructions until reaching the orange level. Once you've gotten there and removed 1 add-on, continue monitoring your weight each week for four more weeks using the table. If your weight shifts from the green zone during the four-week period, refer back to the instructions.

Maintenance week #	Total add-ons	Weight loss over 2 pounds	Weight gain less than 2 pounds	Weight gain 2 pounds or more

When your weight has stayed within the green area for four weeks in a row, you've officially identified your maintenance level! This means you've found the individual level of calories that your body requires to maintain this weight, and you don't need to make any more adjustments to your portion sizes. If you ever feel unsure, you can go back to the table and use it to find your maintenance level again or restart the program from the Set phase if necessary.

Let's take two examples to clarify the add-on system. Angie starts with 1 add-on on week 1. At the end of the week, she weighs herself. She has gained 1 pound (½ kg). Because that falls under the 2-pound (1-kg) mark, she continues to increase her total with 1 add-on and starts week 2 with 2 add-ons. At the end of that week, she weighs herself again. Her weight has remained the same, so she increases her total number of add-ons with 1 more for week 3, totaling 3 add-ons. At the end of week 3, she notices that she has gained 2½ pounds (1¼ kg). She reduces her total number of add-ons from 3 to 2 and continues monitoring her weight for four weeks. If there are no changes to her weight within the 2-pound (1-kg) mark during this period, Angie has found her maintenance level at 2 add-ons.

Daniela kicks off week 1 with 1 add-on. Because of her period, she skips weighing herself at the end of the week and maintains 1 add-on throughout week 2 as well. At the end of week 2, she weighs herself again and has lost 3 pounds (1½ kg) since starting maintenance. She increases her add-ons with 2 for week 3, for a total of 3 add-ons. She steadily continues adding new add-ons for weeks 4, 5, and 6 as her weight remains within the 2-pound (1-kg) mark. At the end of week 6, she has gained 3 pounds (1½ kg) since starting maintenance. She adjusts her total add-ons by reducing 1 for a total of 5 add-ons. If her weight remains stable for four consecutive weeks, Daniela has found her maintenance level at 5 add-ons.

WHAT IF I LOSE TRACK WHILE ON THE MAINTENANCE PLAN AND END UP SKIPPING SEVERAL WEEKS?

Start by weighing yourself. If you've gained more than 5 pounds (2½ kg), return to the Meal Builder for Group 1. Otherwise, stick to the maintenance guidelines.

For example, if you've gained 3 pounds (1½ kg), remove 1 add-on for the following week. If your weight has remained stable within the 2-pound (1-kg) mark, continue your week adding 1 add-on, and if you've lost weight, add 2 add-ons per the instructions.

In this phase, flexibility will be maximized even more. You are now an expert when it comes to portions, know what quantities of different foods are beneficial for your health and feeling great, and have found your ideal meal sizes to keep a steady maintenance level.

Weighing and measuring food has become second nature to you! So much so, that you may want to transition toward a more intuitive way of eating, listening to your body's internal cues, pairing it with the meal building experience you've gained in the previous phase. Because you're now knowledgeable about exactly what goes into your meals, what a balanced plate looks like and what beneficial portion sizes are for you, you can cut back on measuring and weighing ingredients.

For some, the thought of moving away from a structured system that has become so familiar can feel daunting at first. If that's you, try building your meals intuitively one or two days out of the week. Once that feels comfortable, gradually add more days. Measuring and weighing are tools you can always return to when you want to reset, reach a new goal, or remind yourself about portion sizes. To accompany a more flexible way of eating, there's a set of principles that support maintaining your results for life through reinforcing habits that are already familiar to you from previous phases.

the 12 sculpt maintenance tools for life

1 **PRIORITIZE REAL INGREDIENTS**

Choose whole foods over ultra-processed in your daily food choices. When reading food labels in stores, apply what you learned about nutrition in chapter 5 to make well-informed, empowered decisions. Your body will thank you by continuing to function optimally and feeling satisfied after your meals when you keep up with an ideal distribution of each food group.

2 **STICK TO REGULAR MEALTIMES**

Carry on eating breakfast, lunch, dinner, and two snacks per day. Aim to have your breakfast by 9 a.m. and within thirty minutes upon rising, and your last meal by 10 p.m. If you've been on the program for a while, you've probably noticed getting used to your mealtimes and feeling hungry by the four-hour mark. There's a reason for it—on average, the regular stomach has nearly emptied by then. Having structured mealtimes has been shown to have a positive impact on weight, and by continuing to eat frequently, you'll be curbing cravings and avoiding extra snacking in between meals and planned snacks. Stick to your mealtimes to enjoy that steady stream of energy you've been experiencing throughout the program.

3 **ENJOY SPECIAL EVENTS**

One important aspect of the program is balance. Enjoying an evening at a restaurant, a birthday dinner with friends, or a holiday gathering are all memorable, fun parts of a sustainable, balanced lifestyle that you shouldn't miss out on. Remember, what matters is the big picture!

4 **KEEP AHEAD OF HECTIC DAYS**

Your focus has changed from weight loss to maintenance, but your life probably remains just as fast-paced! To keep up with optimal eating, continue planning and cooking your meals ahead of time, freezing some of them for later. You know how much easier life becomes when you plan ahead and stay organized; workdays are hectic enough without having to worry about what you're going to eat.

5 **SWITCH UP YOUR RECIPES**

By now, you've likely found your most-loved recipes that have become everyday staples in your cooking. Explore new recipes and flavors, whether spicy, sweet, or anything in between. This will keep your meals exciting and fun! I hope this program has changed your mindset about healthy food being bland or boring. Keep on testing new ways of seasoning your food, using new spice blends, and trying new dishes. And don't forget to tag your *Sculpt* squad in your food creations at @sculptonline on Instagram! Be sure to visit the website, www.thesculptplan.com, regularly for new recipes, cooking inspiration, ideas, and recommendations.

6 **ALWAYS STAY HYDRATED**

To keep your body hydrated and happy, stick to the habit of drinking water throughout the day by bringing a water bottle with you everywhere you go. Remember that your fluid requirement changes with your weight! Don't forget to update your water goal based on your current weight in pounds by dividing it by 2 to get the daily ounces you should be sipping each day.

7 KEEP IT MOVING

Just like we're going to continue making beneficial food choices, we will also keep up with daily movement! Exercising consistently has a key role in maintaining weight loss in the long run, and evidence even suggests that exercise can help reduce the effect of metabolic adaptation.

You can always push your limits by adding more resistance or pumping up the intensity of your workouts. Continue moving daily and aim to complete higher intensity workouts at least three times a week, combining cardio, weight training, and sculpting sessions. If you feel like changing up your routine or taking your workouts up a notch, all you've got to do is switch to a new program on the app!

8 TRACK YOUR PATH

Track your weight weekly, or at least once a month after you've found your personal maintenance level. Here's why: Monitoring your weight brings awareness to your habits and helps you view your progress over time. In addition to exercise, did you know that keeping track of your weight regularly is one of the strongest evidence-based ways to increase your chances of success in maintaining your happy weight? Whether you log your weight independently or use a digital tool like our app, this simple habit can make a big difference.

9 SET NEW GOALS

Once you are sitting comfortably at your maintenance level, you may feel a desire to set new health goals. For instance, they could include getting stronger or building more lean muscle. Depending on what those goals are, you may need to add more food to your meals to create a caloric surplus. The best way to set and tackle new goals is through the app, where you get a tailored plan with personalized meals and targeted workouts to best fit your new goals.

10 DON'T FORGET SELF-CARE

Sleep, nutrition, movement, and stress management are all essential parts of taking care of your health. All of them are connected to each other, and each one is crucial for your physical and mental well-being. Always remember that self-care is a necessity, not a luxury! When you're busy and stressed, it can become more difficult to prioritize, but putting your needs first does pay off. One of the key takeaways that I hope you've found through this program is that prioritizing yourself is a must for real change to take place. Refer to chapter 9 as often as you need to remind yourself of that!

11 IF YOU FALL, GET BACK UP AGAIN!

If you ever feel the need to start over and return to the weight loss phase, turn back to chapter 3 to refresh your memory about the mindset fundamentals and restart your journey from there. One great aspect about this book is that you can always pick up where you left off. You've done this before, and you've got this!

12 SURROUND YOURSELF WITH SUPPORT

Checking in with your *Sculpt* squad is the best way to stay motivated in maintenance when you've reached this final phase. Inspire new members who are just getting started through your journey, make new friends to cheer each other on, and connect with others who have made it as far as you. Plus, you get access to free workshops and other inspiring members-only events that make continuing this lifestyle easy and fun! If you haven't already, I encourage you to take full advantage of the online bonus parts of the program that are offered to you.

And now we've bittersweetly made it here, all the way to the end of the last chapter. I'm grateful that you've trusted me to guide you through this program. You took the time to learn why certain habits can make a life-changing difference in your journey and applied them into each day. I hope that by the time you're reading this, I've managed to seduce you into a new love for cooking healthy (but so very delicious), timesaving meals. If you haven't yet, explore the recipes on the next pages!

Now that you've reached your happy weight and maintenance level, I trust that you will keep on taking good care of your body and mind. In the meantime, I'll be here for you. We're all in this lifestyle together, for life! Through the app, website, social media, and forthcoming books, my team and I will continue to provide you with access to science-backed resources, flavorful recipes, kitchen tips that maximize convenience along with fresh new updates, so you always have everything you need at your fingertips to maintain the healthy body and life you deserve. I'll see you there!

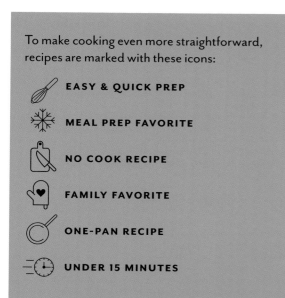

To make cooking even more straightforward, recipes are marked with these icons:

EASY & QUICK PREP

MEAL PREP FAVORITE

NO COOK RECIPE

FAMILY FAVORITE

ONE-PAN RECIPE

UNDER 15 MINUTES

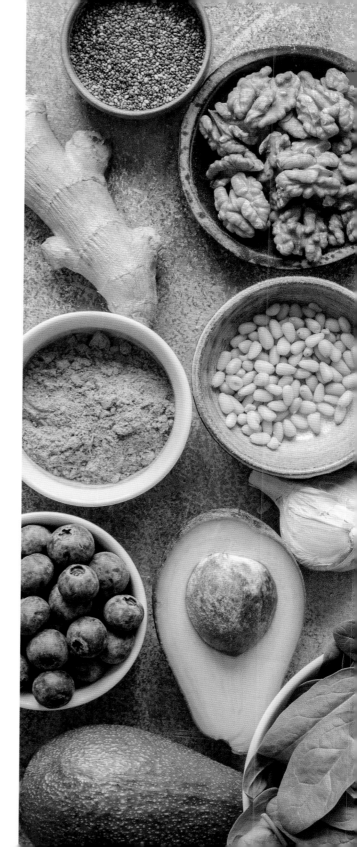

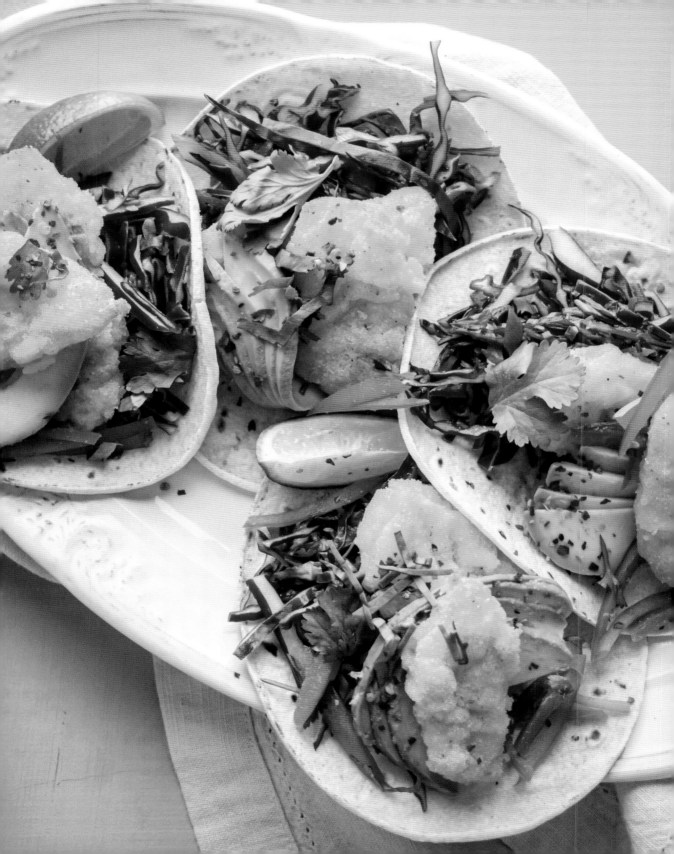

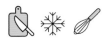

S, GF, V

EASE:
●●○

MAKES:
2 servings

TIME:
6 hours 5 minutes

raspberry almond overnight oats

what you'll need:

GROUP 1

1⅓ cups (265 g) plain nonfat Greek yogurt

⅔ cup (60 g) old-fashioned rolled oats

1 tablespoon (10 g) chia seeds

½ tablespoon (8 g) almond butter

½ teaspoon ground cinnamon

½ teaspoon dry stevia, or more to taste

½ cup (120 ml) unsweetened plain almond milk

1½ cups (190 g) fresh raspberries

GROUP 2

2 cups (400 g) plain nonfat Greek yogurt

⅔ cup (60 g) old-fashioned rolled oats

1 tablespoon (10 g) chia seeds

½ tablespoon (8 g) almond butter

½ teaspoon ground cinnamon

½ teaspoon dry stevia, or more to taste

¼ cup (60 ml) unsweetened plain almond milk

1½ cups (190 g) fresh raspberries

GROUP 3

2 cups (400 g) plain nonfat Greek yogurt

⅔ cup (60 g) old-fashioned rolled oats

1 tablespoon (10 g) chia seeds

1 tablespoon (15 g) almond butter

½ teaspoon ground cinnamon

½ teaspoon dry stevia, or more to taste

¼ cup (60 ml) unsweetened plain almond milk

1½ cups (190 g) fresh raspberries

6 almonds, chopped

1 In a medium container, add the yogurt, oats, chia seeds, almond butter, cinnamon, and stevia. Mix until combined. Stir in the almond milk.

2 Cover the container with a lid or plastic wrap, and place in the fridge overnight. In the morning, uncover, taste, and stir in more stevia if a sweeter flavor is desired.

3 Transfer to a glass or mason jar by placing one-quarter of the oat mixture in the bottom of each glass, followed by one-quarter of the raspberries. Top with a layer of oat mixture, then a layer of raspberries. Sprinkle with chopped almonds if indicated for your group.

anita's tip Overnight oats make one of the easiest, quickest, and tastiest breakfast options with less than 5 minutes of prep time and no cooking required! Store it in the fridge for 3 to 4 days, or 2 to 3 months in the freezer.

BREAKFAST

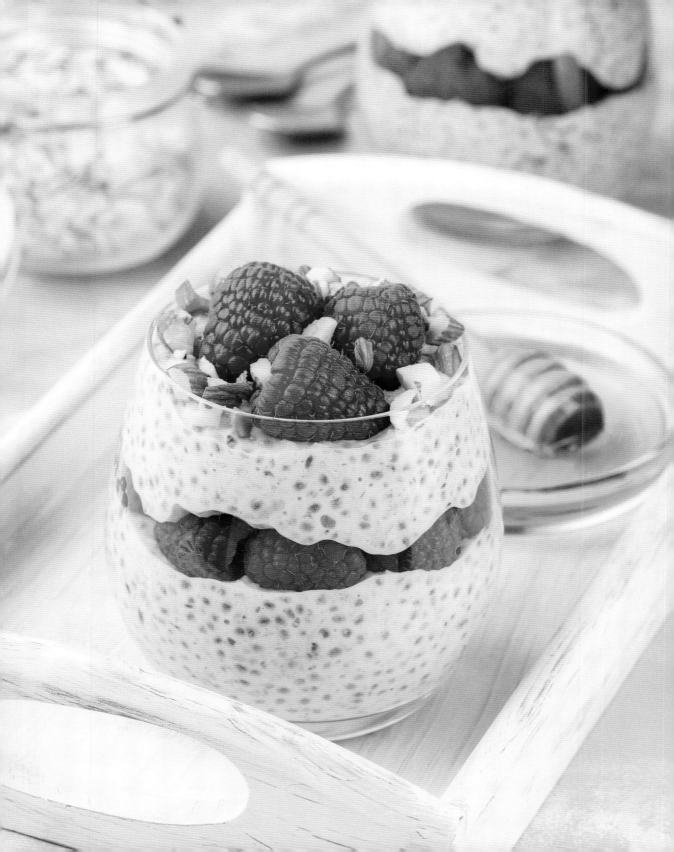

S, GF, V

EASE:
●●○

MAKES:
2 servings

TIME:
35 minutes

chocolatada breakfast bowl

what you'll need:

GROUP 1

2 ounces (60 g) dry quinoa
1 tablespoon (5 g) raw cacao powder
2 tablespoons (15 g) dry stevia
2 cups (475 ml) skim milk, divided
½ small banana, sliced
1 tablespoon (5 g) sliced fresh coconut
⅓ cup (75 g) pomegranate seeds
½ tablespoon (6 g) dark chocolate chips

GROUP 2

2 ounces (60 g) dry quinoa
1 tablespoon (5 g) raw cacao powder
2 tablespoons (15 g) dry stevia
2 cups (475 ml) skim milk, divided
½ small banana, sliced
1 tablespoon (5 g) sliced fresh coconut
⅓ cup (75 g) pomegranate seeds
½ tablespoon (6 g) dark chocolate chips
⅔ cup (135 g) nonfat Greek yogurt, plain or vanilla

GROUP 3

2 ounces (60 g) dry quinoa
1 tablespoon (5 g) raw cacao powder
2 tablespoons (15 g) dry stevia

2 cups (475 ml) skim milk, divided
½ small banana, sliced
3 tablespoons (15 g) sliced fresh coconut
⅓ cup (75 g) pomegranate seeds
1 tablespoon (10 g) dark chocolate chips
⅔ cup (135 g) nonfat Greek yogurt, plain or vanilla

1 Prepare the quinoa by thoroughly rinsing it under cold water in a fine-mesh strainer for 2 to 3 minutes. Drain fully.

2 Heat a small saucepan over medium heat. Add the drained quinoa and toast for 3 minutes, stirring frequently, to slightly toast quinoa and to allow water to evaporate.

3 In a small bowl, combine the cacao powder and stevia. Stir in 1 cup (235 ml) of milk, pouring it little by little while continuing to stir to dissolve larger pieces of cacao. Pour the mixture into the saucepan over the quinoa. Bring to a boil over high heat, then reduce the heat and simmer uncovered for 15 to 20 minutes, stirring occasionally, or until the liquid is fully absorbed and the quinoa is tender. Remove from the heat.

4 Place the chocolate quinoa in two bowls and pour in the remaining milk. Serve with sliced banana, pomegranate seeds, dark chocolate chips, and yogurt, if indicated for your group.

anita's tip Don't skip rinsing quinoa before cooking! Rinsing removes its natural coating, which can have a bitter taste. Some quinoa comes prerinsed, but you can't go wrong with an additional rinse.

BREAKFAST

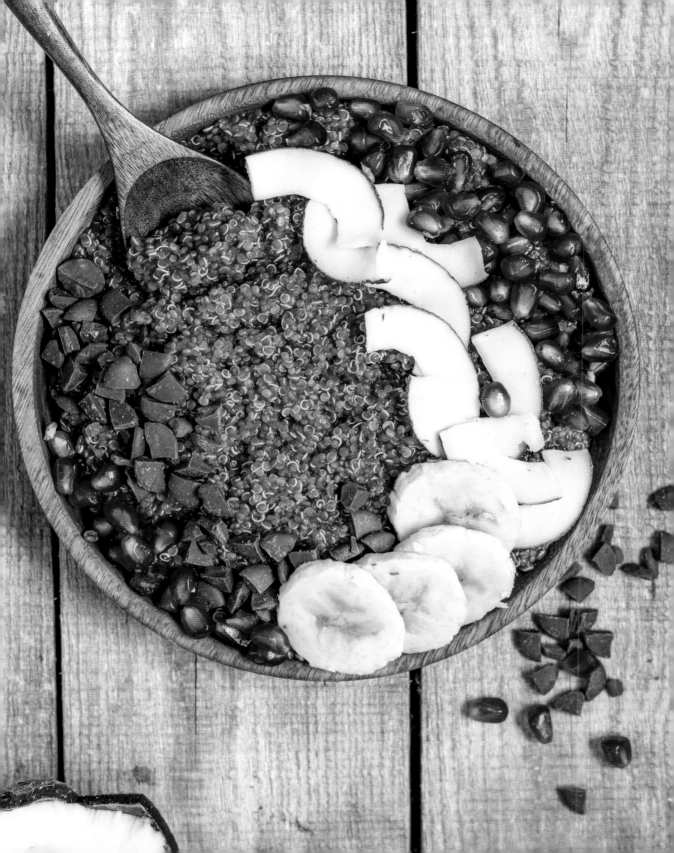

S, GF, V

EASE:
●●●

MAKES:
3 servings

TIME:
2 hours 25 minutes

golden waffle platter with nice cream & nutella

what you'll need:

GROUP 1
Nice cream

1 cup (150 g) sliced very ripe banana, frozen
½ cup (120 ml) unsweetened almond milk, plain

Waffles

4 quick sprays cooking oil
⅔ cup (60 g) old-fashioned rolled oats
2 small eggs
⅔ cup (150 g) low-fat cottage cheese
2 tablespoons (15 g) vanilla protein powder
3 tablespoons (20 g) coconut flour
1 tablespoon (8 g) dry stevia, or more to taste
½ teaspoon baking powder
½ teaspoon pure vanilla extract
Dash of salt
¼ cup (40 g) mixed berries, sliced
1½ tablespoons (25 g) chocolate hazelnut spread (Nutella)

GROUP 2
Nice cream

1 cup (150 g) sliced very ripe banana, frozen
½ cup (120 ml) unsweetened almond milk, plain

Waffles

4 quick sprays cooking oil
⅔ cup (60 g) old-fashioned rolled oats
3 small eggs
⅔ cup (150 g) low-fat cottage cheese
¼ cup (30 g) vanilla protein powder
3 tablespoons (20 g) coconut flour
1 tablespoon (8 g) dry stevia, or more to taste
½ teaspoon baking powder
½ teaspoon pure vanilla extract
Dash of salt
¼ cup (40 g) mixed berries, sliced
1½ tablespoons (25 g) chocolate hazelnut spread (Nutella)

GROUP 3
Nice cream

1 cup (150 g) sliced very ripe banana, frozen
½ cup (120 ml) unsweetened almond milk, plain

Waffles

4 quick sprays cooking oil
⅔ cup (60 g) old-fashioned rolled oats
3 small eggs
⅔ cup (150 g) low-fat cottage cheese
¼ cup (30 g) vanilla protein powder
3 tablespoons (20 g) coconut flour
1 tablespoon (8 g) dry stevia, or more to taste
½ teaspoon baking powder
½ teaspoon pure vanilla extract
Dash of salt
¼ cup (40 g) mixed berries, sliced
3 tablespoons (50 g) chocolate hazelnut spread (Nutella)

BREAKFAST

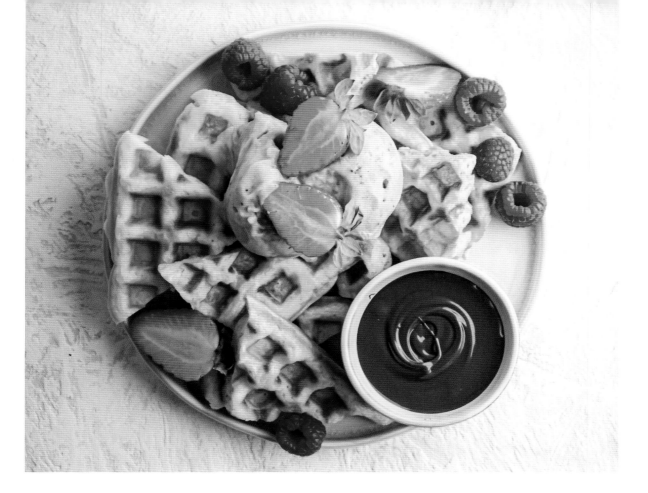

1 To make the nice cream, add the banana and almond milk to a blender. Mix for 1 minute. If you're having a hard time reaching a purée-like consistency, add more almond milk. Return to the freezer for 2 hours, or until it reaches an ice cream-like consistency.

2 To make the waffles, preheat a waffle iron to medium-high heat. Lightly coat with 4 quick sprays of cooking oil.

3 In a blender, grind the oats into flour. Add the eggs, cottage cheese, protein powder, coconut flour, stevia, baking powder, vanilla, and salt. Blend until smooth. Pour a thin layer of the mixture onto the waffle iron, close gently and cook until golden brown and crisp, about 4 to 5 minutes.

4 To serve, cut the waffles into pieces. Remove the banana nice cream from the freezer. Scoop a ball on top of the waffle platter and serve with Nutella.

anita's tip Instead of nice cream, you can slice the banana and serve it with the berries. Use Nutella as a dip, or drizzle on top. The flavor of coconut oil cooking spray goes great with this recipe!

sweet potato chorizo ham frittata

what you'll need:

GROUP 1

4 small eggs

½ cup (120 ml) unsweetened almond milk, plain

½ teaspoon salt

¼ teaspoon ground black pepper

1 tablespoon (3 g) finely chopped fresh chives

¼ cup (30 g) shredded cheddar cheese, divided

2 teaspoons (10 ml) extra-virgin olive oil

1½ ounces (45 g) chorizo sausage, skin removed and roughly chopped

1½ ounces (45 g) smoked deli ham, roughly chopped

½ small yellow onion, finely chopped

3½ cups (450 g) peeled and diced sweet potato

2 cloves garlic, minced

GROUP 2

5 small eggs

½ cup (120 ml) unsweetened almond milk, plain

½ teaspoon salt

¼ teaspoon ground black pepper

1 tablespoon (3 g) finely chopped fresh chives

¼ cup (30 g) shredded cheddar cheese, divided

2 teaspoons (10 ml) extra-virgin olive oil

2½ ounces (70 g) chorizo sausage, skin removed and roughly chopped

3 ounces (85 g) smoked deli ham, roughly chopped

½ small yellow onion, finely chopped

3½ cups (450 g) peeled and diced sweet potato

2 cloves garlic, minced

GROUP 3

5 small eggs

½ cup (120 ml) unsweetened almond milk, plain

½ teaspoon salt

¼ teaspoon ground black pepper

1 tablespoon (3 g) finely chopped fresh chives

½ cup (60 g) shredded cheddar cheese, divided

4 teaspoons (20 ml) extra-virgin olive oil

2 ½ ounces (70 g) chorizo sausage, skin removed and roughly chopped

3 ounces (85 g) ham, roughly chopped

½ small yellow onion, finely chopped

3½ cups (450 g) peeled and diced sweet potato

2 cloves garlic, minced

1 Preheat the oven to 375°F (190°C). Break the eggs into a medium mixing bowl. Add the almond milk, salt, pepper, chives, and half of the shredded cheese, whisking until smooth. Set aside.

2 Heat the oil in a large, ovenproof, nonstick skillet over medium-high heat. Add the chorizo, ham, and onion. Cook until the onion is softened and the chorizo is completely cooked through, about 4 minutes. Add the sweet potato and garlic to the pan. Continue frying for 2 minutes. Pour in the egg mixture and cook for about 5 minutes, or until partially set.

3 Place the pan in the oven and bake for 10 to 12 minutes. Remove from the oven and sprinkle the remaining shredded cheese over the eggs. Place the skillet back in the oven and bake until the cheese softens and the eggs firm up,

BREAKFAST

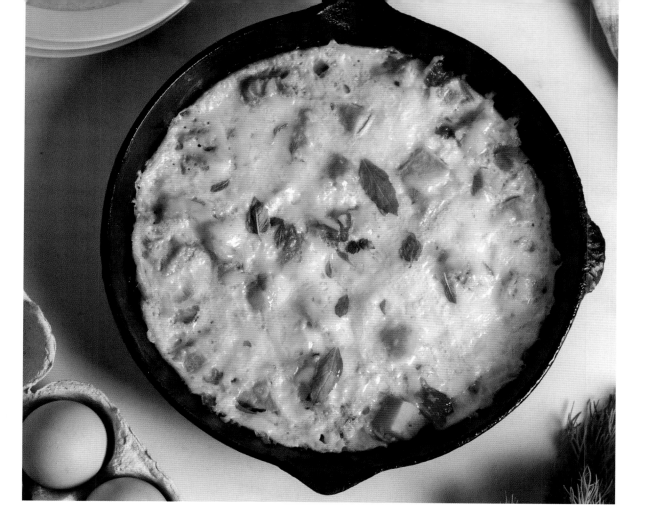

about 5 minutes. If the middle still wobbles, it needs a little longer in the oven.

4 Let stand for a few minutes before cutting. Serve warm or at room temperature.

NOTE: *To complete your breakfast, add 1 portion of fruit as dessert.*

DF: *To make this recipe dairy-free, replace the shredded cheddar with plant-based cheese shreds.*

anita's tip A frittata is an open-faced omelet that gives you endless possibilities. Throw in any non-starchy vegetables, like mushrooms, peppers, asparagus, or tomatoes. Not a big fan of sweet potatoes? Swap for white potatoes!

S, GF, V

 EASE:
●○○

MAKES:
1 serving

 TIME:
5 minutes

dark chocolate pudding cup

what you'll need:

GROUP 1

⅔ cup (135 g) nonfat Greek yogurt, plain or vanilla

2 tablespoons (10 g) raw cacao powder

2 teaspoons (14 g) honey

½ teaspoon dry stevia

¼ cup (30 g) granola

GROUP 2

1 cup (200 g) nonfat Greek yogurt, plain or vanilla, divided

2 tablespoons (10 g) raw cacao powder

2 teaspoons (14 g) honey

½ teaspoon dry stevia

¼ cup (30 g) granola

GROUP 3

1 cup (200 g) nonfat Greek yogurt, plain or vanilla, divided

2 tablespoons (10 g) raw cacao powder

2 teaspoons (14 g) honey

1 teaspoon dry stevia

¼ cup (30 g) granola

½ tablespoon (6 g) dark chocolate chips

1 In a small bowl, combine ⅔ cup (135 g) yogurt, cacao powder, honey, and stevia with 1 tablespoon (15 ml) of water until reaching a pudding-like consistency. Add more water if the mixture is too thick for the ingredients to mix well. Transfer the mixture to a glass. For groups 2 and 3, top with remaining yogurt.

2 Sprinkle the pudding with granola (and dark chocolate chips for group 3) and serve.

NOTE: *To complete your breakfast, add 1 portion of fruit as dessert.*

anita's tip Made with rich raw cacao, the superfood of all superfoods, these cups are guaranteed to satisfy your sweet tooth! Raw cacao is packed with antioxidants, magnesium, and calcium. The sweeter you prefer it, the more stevia you can add; a little goes a long way, so taste as you go.

S, GF

EASE:
●●○

MAKES:
1 serving

TIME:
30 minutes

easy turkey, cheese & egg pockets

what you'll need:

GROUP 1

4 quick sprays cooking oil

1 (6-inch [15-cm]) tortilla wrap of choice

1 small egg

2 slices smoked deli turkey

2 tablespoons (15 g) shredded cheddar cheese

GROUP 2

4 quick sprays cooking oil

1 (6-inch [15-cm]) tortilla wrap of choice

1 small egg

4 slices smoked deli turkey

2 tablespoons (15 g) shredded cheddar cheese

GROUP 3

4 quick sprays cooking oil

1 (6-inch [15-cm]) tortilla wrap of choice

1 small egg

4 slices smoked deli turkey

¼ cup (30 g) shredded cheddar cheese

1   Preheat the oven to 375°F (190°C). Place a large piece of foil on a cutting board, spray the foil with cooking spray, and place the tortilla flat on it. Place the turkey slices flat in the middle of the tortilla. Add the cheddar in the middle of the turkey, leaving an empty circle in the middle. Crack an egg in the middle of the circle.

2   Working at a quick pace, fold the bottom and top edges of the tortilla in, then the left and right side to form a tight pocket. Wrap in the foil without turning the pocket upside down as the egg can leak.

3   Place the foil pocket in the oven and bake for 20 to 25 minutes. The base and edges should be crispy and the top will be soft when you open the foil. When done, unwrap from foil and immediately cut in half to serve.

NOTE: *To complete your breakfast, add 1 portion of fruit as dessert.*

DF: *To make this recipe dairy-free, replace shredded cheddar with plant-based cheddar-style shreds.*

anita's tip Use this freezer-friendly recipe as a base for your own creations! You can swap smoked turkey for any protein of your choice, such as turkey bacon, ham, chorizo, or meatless crumbles. Both white flour tortillas and whole wheat tortillas go amazingly with these pockets!

S, GF, V

EASE:
●●○

MAKES:
2 servings

TIME:
20 minutes

creamy tropical summer oatmeal

what you'll need:

GROUP 1

1 tablespoon (15 g) unsalted butter
⅔ cup (60 g) old-fashioned rolled oats
1 cup (235 ml) skim milk
1 tablespoon (7 g) vanilla protein powder
½ teaspoon ground cinnamon, or more to taste
Pinch of salt
⅓ cup (75 g) low-fat cottage cheese
¼ small orange
⅓ small banana
½ cup (85 g) cubed fresh mango

GROUP 2

1 tablespoon (15 g) unsalted butter
⅔ cup (60 g) old-fashioned rolled oats
1 cup (235 ml) skim milk
3 tablespoons (20 g) vanilla protein powder
½ teaspoon ground cinnamon, or more to taste
Pinch of salt
⅓ cup (75 g) low-fat cottage cheese
¼ small orange
⅓ small banana
½ cup (85 g) cubed fresh mango

GROUP 3

2 tablespoons (30 g) unsalted butter
⅔ cup (60 g) old-fashioned rolled oats
1 cup (235 ml) skim milk
3 tablespoons (20 g) vanilla protein powder
½ teaspoon ground cinnamon, or more to taste
Pinch of salt
⅓ cup (75 g) low-fat cottage cheese
¼ small orange
⅓ small banana
½ cup (85 g) cubed fresh mango

1 Melt the butter in a small saucepan over medium heat. Once melted, add the oats and stir to coat. Cook, stirring occasionally, until the oats smell toasty, about 4 to 6 minutes.

2 Pour in the milk, and add the protein powder, cinnamon, and salt. Reduce the heat to low and let simmer uncovered, stirring occasionally until the oats are soft and fluffy, and have absorbed most of the liquid, about 8 to 10 minutes. If the oats absorb the milk quickly, add water as needed. Remove from the heat, add the cottage cheese, cover, and let stand for 2 to 3 minutes.

3 In the meantime, peel and slice the orange and banana. Transfer the oatmeal to two bowls and top with fruit.

anita's tip Leftover oatmeal will stay good in the fridge for about 4 days. To store, let it cool to room temperature, then cover and refrigerate. Top with fresh fruit every morning when serving!

BREAKFAST

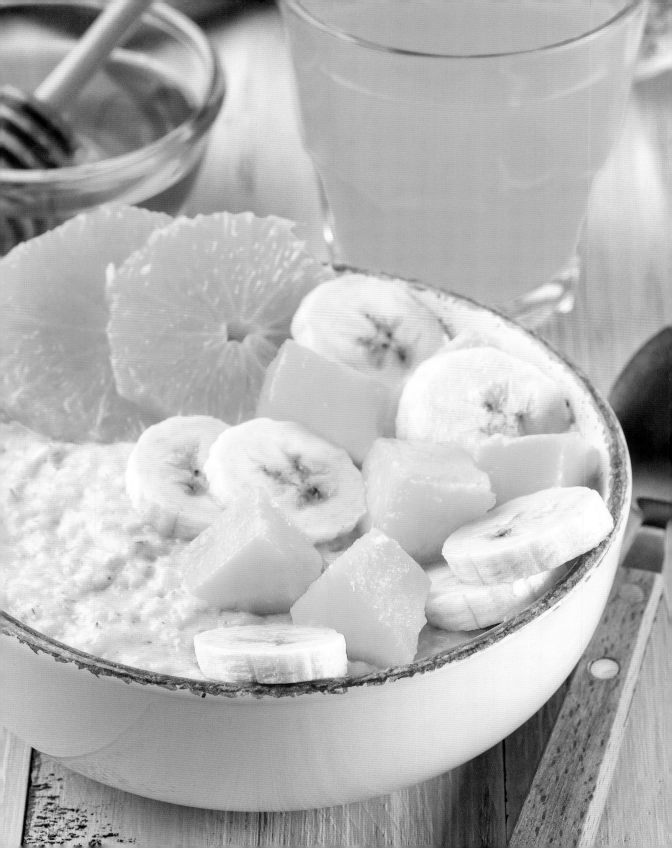

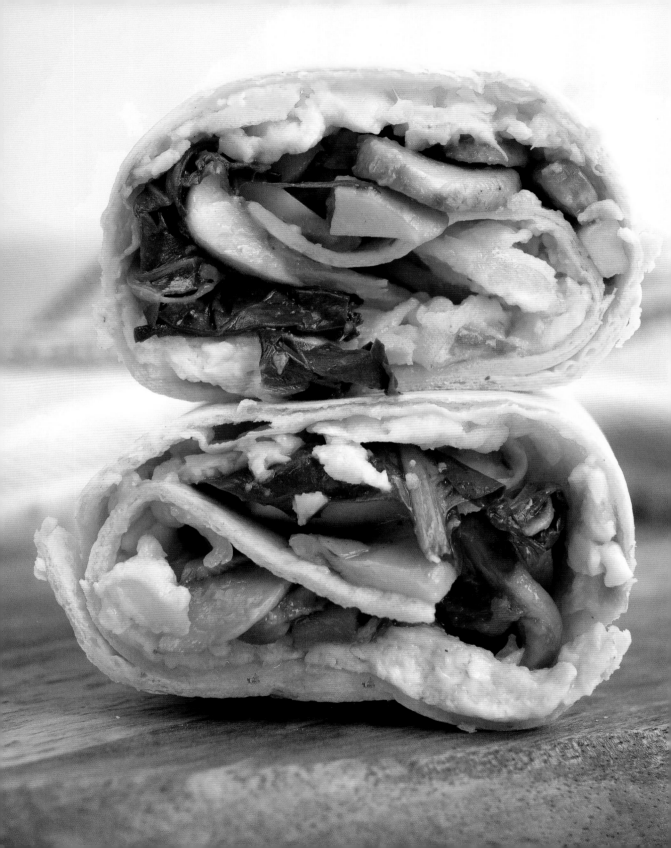

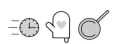

S, GF, V

EASE:
●●○

MAKES:
2 servings

TIME:
15 minutes

cheesy mushroom omelet wraps

what you'll need:

GROUP 1

2 (6-inch [15-cm]) tortilla wraps of choice

1 teaspoon extra-virgin olive oil

1 cup (100 g) baby bella mushrooms, sliced

1 cup (55 g) baby spinach, roughly chopped

4 small eggs

¼ teaspoon salt

⅛ teaspoon ground black pepper

2 tablespoons (15 g) shredded Swiss cheese

GROUP 2

2 (6-inch [15-cm]) tortilla wraps of choice

1 teaspoon extra-virgin olive oil

1 cup (100 g) baby bella mushrooms, sliced

1 cup (55 g) baby spinach, roughly chopped

6 small eggs

¼ teaspoon salt

⅛ teaspoon ground black pepper

2 tablespoons (15 g) shredded Swiss cheese

GROUP 3

2 (6-inch [15-cm]) tortilla wraps of choice

2 teaspoons (10 ml) extra-virgin olive oil

1 cup (100 g) baby bella mushrooms, sliced

1 cup (55 g) baby spinach, roughly chopped

6 small eggs

¼ teaspoon salt

⅛ teaspoon ground black pepper

¼ cup (30 g) shredded Swiss cheese

1 Heat the tortilla wraps in a medium nonstick skillet over medium heat, no more than 30 seconds per side. Set the tortillas on a plate.

2 In the same skillet, heat the oil over medium heat. Add the mushrooms and cook for 4 to 5 minutes until browned. Add the spinach and cook for 2 to 3 minutes until wilted. Set aside.

3 Crack the eggs in the skillet. Using a fork to break the yolks,

lightly scramble the egg mixture. Season with salt and pepper.

4 Spread the scrambled egg mixture on each tortilla. Top with cheese, then add mushrooms and spinach. Roll up the wraps burrito-style and cut in half.

NOTE: *To complete your breakfast, have 1 portion of fruit as dessert.*

DF: *To make this recipe dairy-free, replace Swiss cheese with plant-based Swiss-style slices.*

anita's tip Not a lover of Swiss cheese? Any melting cheese, from cheddar and part-skim mozzarella to Parmesan and plant-based cheese shreds will work great with this recipe.

S, GF, V

EASE:

● ○ ○

MAKES:
2 servings

TIME:

10 minutes

strawberry banana chia smoothie bowl

what you'll need:

GROUP 1
⅔ cup (60 g) old-fashioned rolled oats
1⅓ cups (265 g) nonfat Greek yogurt,
   plain
1 cup (170 g) sliced fresh strawberries
½ small banana, sliced
1 tablespoon (10 g) chia seeds
1 tablespoon (5 g) almonds, chopped

GROUP 2
⅔ cup (60 g) old-fashioned rolled oats
2 cups (400 g) nonfat Greek yogurt,
   plain
1 cup (170 g) sliced fresh strawberries
½ small banana, sliced
1 tablespoon (10 g) chia seeds
1 tablespoon (5 g) almonds, chopped

GROUP 3
⅔ cup (60 g) old-fashioned rolled oats
2 cups (400 g) nonfat Greek yogurt,
   plain
1 cup (170 g) sliced fresh strawberries
½ small banana, sliced
1 tablespoon (10 g) chia seeds
3 tablespoons (20 g) almonds,
   chopped

1 Add the oats to your blender. Process until you reach a flour-like consistency.

2 Slice the strawberries and add about three-quarters to the blender with the Greek yogurt. Blend until a thick and creamy smoothie is formed.

3 Transfer the smoothie mixture to a bowl. Add the banana slices on one side of the bowl along with the rest of the strawberry slices.

4 Sprinkle chia seeds and almond pieces in a diagonal line in the middle of the bowl.

anita's tip To switch it up and try different flavors, you can replace chia seeds with unsweetened coconut shreds. Similarly, try swapping strawberry and banana for pineapple, mango, passion fruit, or any other fruit you love!

BREAKFAST

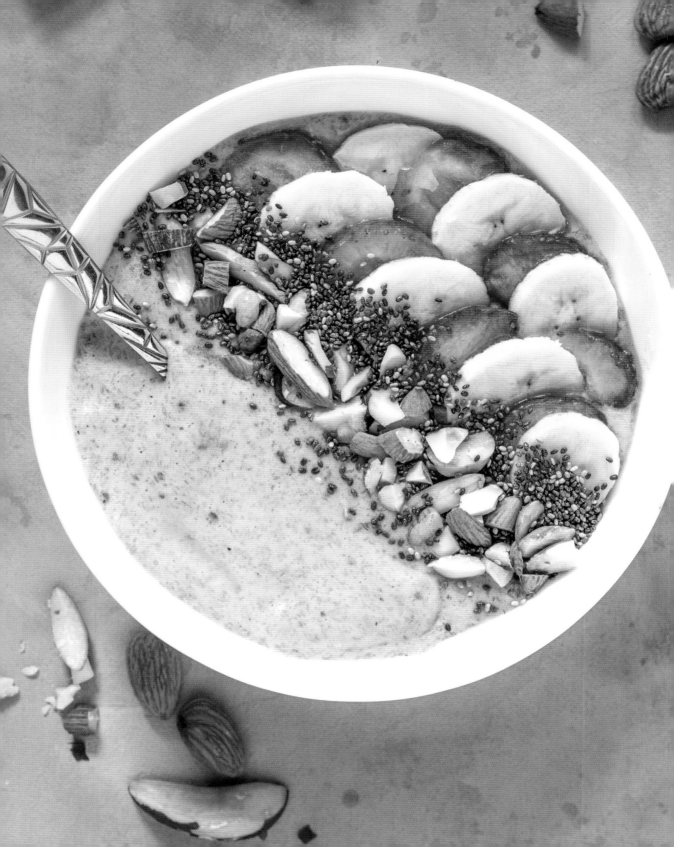

S, DF

EASE:
●●●

MAKES:
2 servings

TIME:
30 minutes

one-pan cajun shrimp penne

what you'll need:

GROUP 1

15 ounces (425 g) raw large shrimp, peeled and deveined

2 teaspoons (5 g) Cajun seasoning (page 84), divided, plus more to taste

2 teaspoons (10 ml) extra-virgin olive oil, divided

1 cup (100 g) mushrooms, sliced

1 bell pepper, thinly sliced

½ cup (65 g) diced yellow onion

1½ cups (355 ml) unsweetened almond milk, plain

1 tablespoon (15 g) almond butter

1 tablespoon (15 ml) low-sodium soy sauce

1 teaspoon liquid smoke

1 cup (235 ml) low-sodium or unsalted chicken broth

3 ounces (85 g) dry penne pasta

½ cup (90 g) canned diced tomatoes, fire-roasted or regular

¼ cup (15 g) finely chopped fresh parsley, optional

GROUPS 2 & 3

1¼ lb. (565 g) raw large shrimp, peeled and deveined

1 tablespoon (8 g) Cajun seasoning (page 84), divided, plus more to taste

2 teaspoons (10 ml) extra-virgin olive oil, divided

1 cup (70 g) sliced mushrooms

1 bell pepper, thinly sliced

½ cup (65 g) diced yellow onion

1½ cups (355 ml) unsweetened almond milk, plain

1 tablespoon (15 g) almond butter

1 tablespoon (15 ml) low-sodium soy sauce

1 teaspoon liquid smoke

1 cup (235 ml) low-sodium or unsalted chicken broth

4 ounces (115 g) dry penne pasta

½ cup (90 g) canned diced tomatoes, fire-roasted or regular

¼ cup (15 g) finely chopped fresh parsley, optional

1 Season the shrimp with one teaspoon of Cajun seasoning.

2 Heat half of the oil in a large, nonstick skillet over medium-high heat. Once the pan is hot, add the shrimp and cook 2 to 3 minutes per side, or until opaque. Transfer the shrimp to a plate.

3 Add the rest of the oil to the skillet. Add the mushrooms, bell pepper, and onion. Sprinkle with the remaining teaspoon of Cajun seasoning. Cook over medium-high until vegetables become tender, about 5 to 6 minutes.

4 In a large bowl, combine the almond milk, almond butter, soy sauce, liquid smoke, and half of the broth. Whisk until smooth. Add to the skillet with the vegetables and bring the mixture to a boil.

5 Once boiling, add the dry penne. Cover and reduce the heat to medium. Simmer for 10 to 12 minutes, or until the pasta is al dente.

6 Meanwhile, add the diced tomatoes to a blender. Blend well.

LUNCH

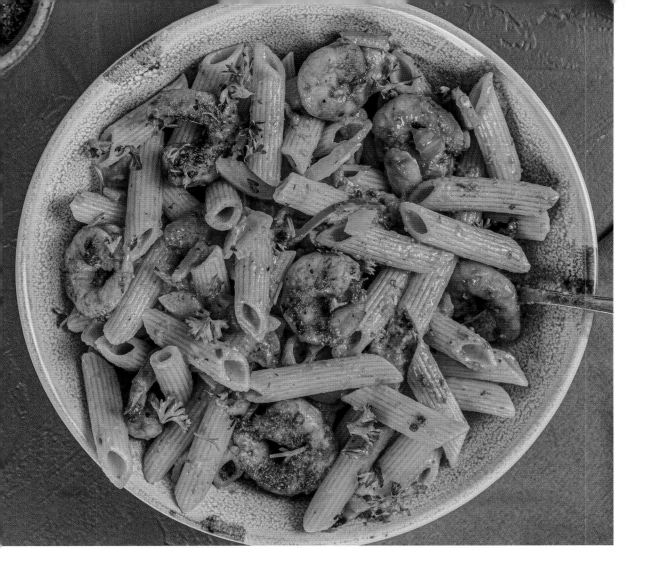

7   Uncover the pasta and stir in the tomato liquid
    and remaining broth. Bring the sauce to a boil.
    Stir in the shrimp and fresh parsley, if using, taste,
    and add more Cajun seasoning if desired.

anita's tip The amount of Cajun seasoning provided in the recipe is great if you're into
the Cajun flavor but prefer it mild. If you're
looking to turn up the heat, add more seasoning
in step 3. Use the homemade Cajun seasoning
(page 84). Most store-bought ones come with
added salt, which paired with soy sauce would
make this dish way too salty!

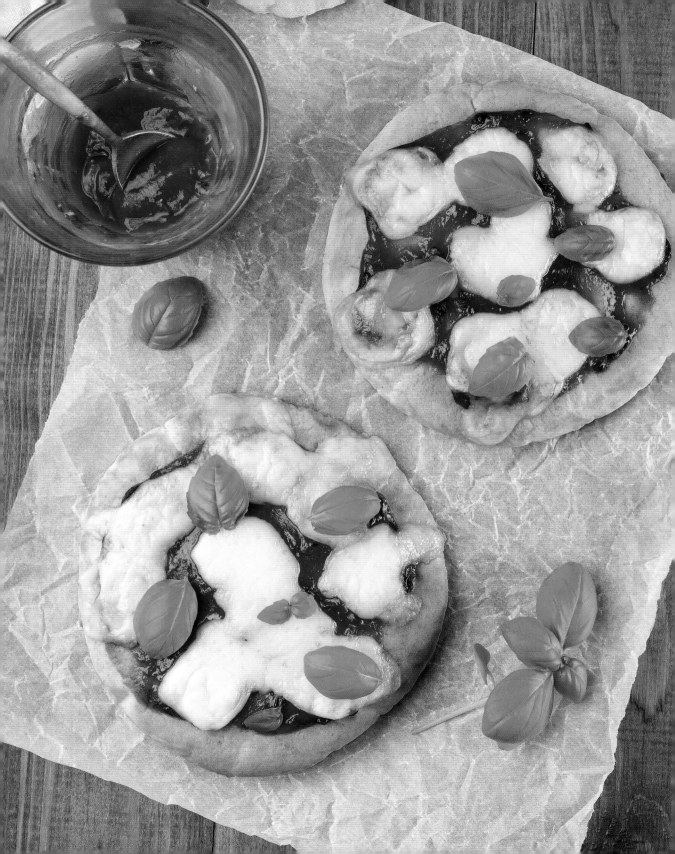

margherita mini pita pizzas

what you'll need:

GROUP 1

1 serving = 1½ pizzas

3 small (4-inch [10-cm]) pita breads (pitettes)

3 tablespoons (45 ml) tomato sauce

4 teaspoons (20 ml) extra-virgin olive oil

3 ounces (85 g) mozzarella cheese, part-skim

¼ teaspoon garlic powder

¼ teaspoon dried oregano

Fresh basil, optional

GROUPS 2 & 3

1 serving = 2 pizzas

4 small (4-inch [10-cm]) pita breads (pitettes)

¼ cup (60 ml) tomato sauce

4 teaspoons (20 ml) extra-virgin olive oil

4 ounces (115 g) mozzarella cheese, part-skim

¼ teaspoon garlic powder

¼ teaspoon dried oregano

Fresh basil, optional

1 Preheat the oven to 400°F (200°C). In a small mixing bowl, combine the tomato sauce and oil.

2 Place the pita breads on a baking sheet and brush sauce on each. Evenly divide the cheese over top. Bake until the cheese is melted and golden brown, about 10 to 12 minutes.

3 Top with garlic powder, dried oregano, and fresh basil if using.

anita's tip Looking to add toppings? Add all the non-starchy veggies you like from the unlimited list, such as sliced mushroom or bell peppers. You can also borrow protein or fruit portions from other meals of the day to add your favorite toppings.

air-fryer crispy chicken nuggets & honey mustard dip

what you'll need:

GROUP 1
Nuggets

6¼ ounces (175 g) uncooked chicken breast, skinless and boneless
⅓ cup (30 g) old-fashioned rolled oats
3 tablespoons (20 g) coconut flour
2 tablespoons (10 g) grated Parmesan cheese
1 tablespoon (3 g) Italian Seasoning (page 85)
½ teaspoon salt
¼ teaspoon ground black pepper
1 teaspoon smoked paprika
¼ teaspoon garlic powder
1 small egg, beaten
Cooking oil spray

Honey Mustard Dip

3 tablespoons (40 g) low-fat mayonnaise
1 tablespoon (15 g) Dijon mustard
2 teaspoons (15 g) honey
½ teaspoon apple cider vinegar

GROUPS 2 & 3
Nuggets

8¾ ounces (250 g) uncooked chicken breast, skinless and boneless
⅓ cup (30 g) old-fashioned rolled oats
⅓ cup (40 g) coconut flour
2 tablespoons (10 g) grated Parmesan cheese
1 tablespoon (3 g) Italian seasoning (page 85)
½ teaspoon salt, divided
¼ teaspoon ground black pepper, divided
1 teaspoon smoked paprika
¼ teaspoon garlic powder
1 small egg, beaten
Cooking oil spray

Honey Mustard Dip

3 tablespoons (40 g) low-fat mayonnaise
1 tablespoon (15 g) Dijon mustard
2 teaspoons (15 g) honey
½ teaspoon apple cider vinegar

1 To make the nuggets, preheat an air fryer to 400°F (200°C). Dice the chicken breast into nugget-size bites and set on a plate.

2 Blend the oats in a blender or food processor until it resembles flour. Add the coconut flour, Parmesan, Italian seasoning, salt, pepper, garlic powder, and smoked paprika, and mix.

3 Place the oat mixture on a plate or shallow bowl. On a second plate or bowl, add the beaten egg.

4 Spray the air-fryer basket lightly with oil. One by one, dip each piece of chicken in the seasoned flour-like oat mixture, then in the egg, and then back in the flour. Place the chicken in the air fryer, and coat again lightly with oil. Cook for about 12 to 14 minutes, or until golden and crispy, turning halfway through the cooking time.

LUNCH

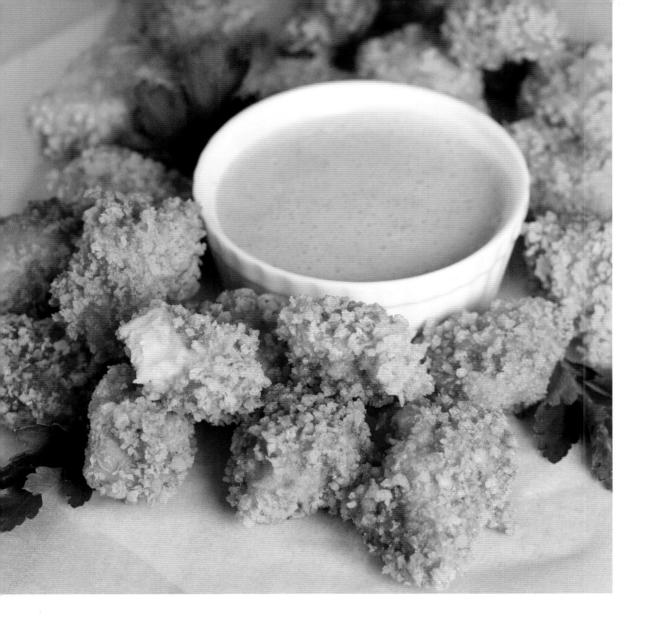

5　To make the honey mustard dip, mix the mayonnaise, Dijon mustard, honey, and apple cider vinegar in a small dish. Serve with the nuggets and a side of fresh or steamed vegetables.

NOTE: *Serve with ½ portion starch of choice per serving, or alternatively roll it over to another meal.*

anita's tip This one takes a little more extra effort than most of the recipes in this book, but trust me, it's one of those dishes that always have everyone asking, *"Can this really be healthy?"*

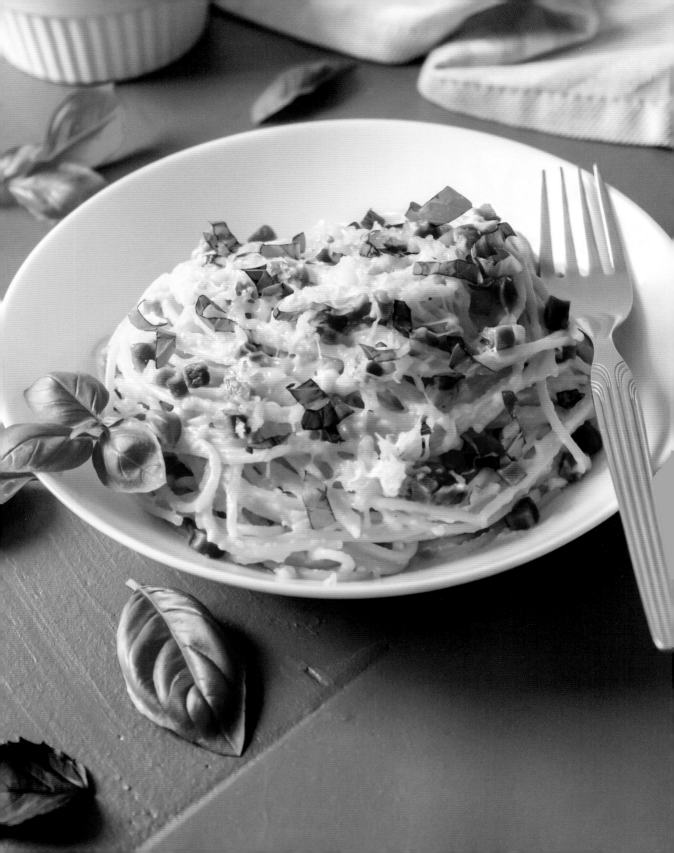

S, GF

 EASE:
●●○

 MAKES:
1 serving

 TIME:
50 minutes

italian-style pasta carbonara

what you'll need:

GROUP 1

1½ ounces (45 g) dry spaghetti of choice

1 small egg

2 tablespoons (10 g) grated Parmesan
    cheese

½ tablespoon (7 g) unsalted butter

4 slices turkey bacon, chopped

2 cloves garlic, minced

¼ teaspoon salt

⅛ teaspoon ground black pepper

1 tablespoon (4 g) finely chopped fresh
    parsley

GROUPS 2 & 3

2 ounces (60 g) dry spaghetti of choice

1 small egg

2 tablespoons (10 g) grated Parmesan
    cheese

½ tablespoon (7 g) unsalted butter

6 slices turkey bacon, chopped

2 cloves garlic, minced

¼ teaspoon salt

⅛ teaspoon ground black pepper

1 tablespoon (4 g) finely chopped fresh
    parsley

1   Take the egg out of the fridge to room temperature
    30 minutes before cooking.

2   In a large pot of boiling water, cook the spaghetti according
    to package instructions. Drain well, and reserve ¼ cup
    (60 ml) of cooking water.

3   In a small bowl, whisk together the egg yolk and Parmesan.
    Set aside.

4   Heat the butter on a medium, nonstick skillet over medi-
    um-high heat. Add the turkey bacon and cook until brown
    and crispy, about 5 to 10 minutes depending on how crispy
    you like your bacon. Stir in the garlic and cook until fra-
    grant, about 1 minute. Remove the skillet from the heat.

5   Working quickly, add the pasta, toss, and stir in the egg mix-
    ture. The pasta should be hot for the egg to cook, but not
    too hot where it becomes scrambled. Toss to combine. Add
    some reserved spaghetti cooking water 1 tablespoon (15 ml)
    at a time, if needed, until a creamy consistency is reached.
    Season with salt and pepper. Top with parsley and serve.

anita's tip If you like your turkey bacon very crispy,
try making it in the air fryer! Pop it in for 10 to 12 minutes at
380°F (195°C).

LUNCH

greek-style tzatziki chicken wraps

what you'll need:

GROUP 1

1 serving = 1½ wraps

6¼ ounces (175 g) uncooked chicken breast, skinless and boneless

1 tablespoon (15 ml) fresh lemon juice, divided

4 teaspoons (20 ml) extra-virgin olive oil, divided

½ teaspoon dried oregano

½ teaspoon salt, divided

¼ teaspoon ground black pepper, divided

½ small cucumber, deseeded and grated

⅓ cup (65 g) plain nonfat Greek yogurt

1 small clove garlic, finely minced

½ teaspoon dried dill

¼ teaspoon dried mint, optional

3 (6-inch [15-cm]) tortilla wraps of choice

½ small bell pepper, sliced

/2 cup (75 g) cherry tomatoes, halved

½ cup (30 g) shredded lettuce

GROUPS 2 & 3

1 serving = 2 wraps

8¾ ounces (250 g) uncooked chicken breast, skinless and boneless

1 tablespoon (15 ml) fresh lemon juice, divided

4 teaspoons (20 ml) extra-virgin olive oil, divided

½ teaspoon dried oregano

½ teaspoon salt, divided

¼ teaspoon ground black pepper, divided

½ small cucumber, deseeded and grated

⅓ cup (65 g) plain nonfat Greek yogurt

1 small clove garlic, finely minced

½ teaspoon dried dill

¼ teaspoon dried mint, optional

4 (6-inch [15-cm]) tortilla wraps of choice

½ cup (30 g) shredded lettuce

½ cup (75 g) cherry tomatoes, halved

½ small bell pepper, sliced

1 Place the chicken breast in a bowl. Add half a tablespoon (8 ml) of lemon juice, 1 teaspoon of oil, and the oregano. Season with half of salt and pepper. Toss and set aside to marinate for at least 15 minutes.

2 To make the tzatziki sauce, place the cucumber, yogurt, garlic, dill, mint (if using), remaining lemon juice, and 2 teaspoons (10 ml) of oil in a small bowl. Season with remaining salt and pepper and mix well.

3 Heat the remaining 1 teaspoon of oil in a medium, nonstick skillet over medium-high heat. Add the chicken breast and cook until both sides are golden and cook through, about 2 to 3 minutes per side. Transfer the chicken to a plate and let stand for about 5 minutes before cutting into smaller pieces.

4 Place each tortilla on a flat surface, spread about 1 heaped tablespoon (15 to 20 ml) of tzatziki sauce over it, top with a couple of chicken pieces, bell pepper, tomatoes, and lettuce. Roll up the wrap. Repeat with the remaining tortillas.

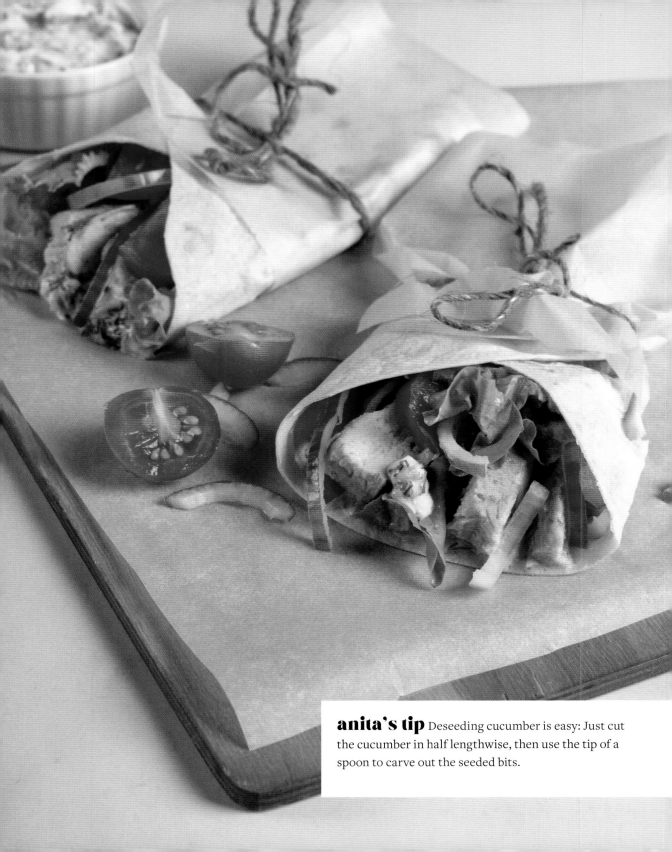

anita's tip Deseeding cucumber is easy: Just cut the cucumber in half lengthwise, then use the tip of a spoon to carve out the seeded bits.

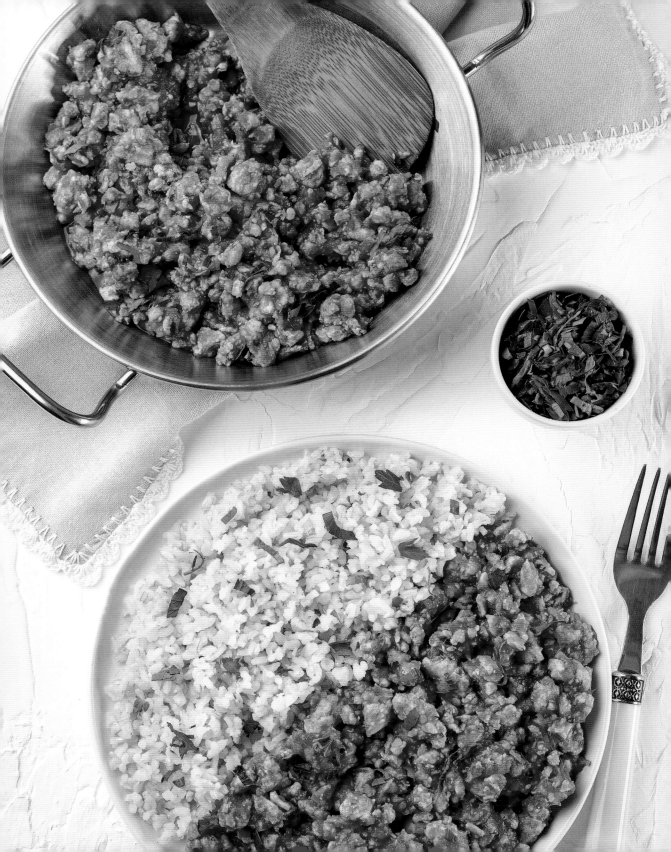

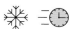 **S, DF, GF**

EASE:
●●○

MAKES:
2 servings

TIME:
25 minutes

cuban-style turkey picadillo

what you'll need:

GROUP 1

3 ounces (85 g) dry brown rice, well rinsed

1 tablespoon (15 ml) extra-virgin olive oil, divided

7½ ounces (215 g) uncooked lean ground turkey, 93%

¼ teaspoon salt

⅛ teaspoon ground black pepper

½ small yellow onion, finely chopped

2 cloves garlic, minced

1 red bell pepper, sliced

½ cup (90 g) canned diced tomatoes

8 green olives plus 1 tablespoon (15 ml) brine

½ teaspoon ground cumin

1 bay leaf

1 tablespoon (1 g) finely chopped fresh cilantro, optional

GROUPS 2 & 3

4 ounces (115 g) dry brown rice, well rinsed

1 tablespoon (15 ml) extra-virgin olive oil

10 ounces (285 g) uncooked lean ground turkey, 93%

¼ teaspoon salt

⅛ teaspoon ground black pepper

½ small yellow onion, finely chopped

2 cloves garlic, minced

1 red bell pepper, sliced

½ cup (90 g) canned diced tomatoes

8 green olives plus 1 tablespoon (15 ml) brine

½ teaspoon ground cumin

1 bay leaf

1 tablespoon (1 g) finely chopped fresh cilantro, optional

1   Prepare the rice according to the package directions. Fluff with a fork and set aside.

2   Heat the oil in a large, nonstick skillet over medium-high heat. Add the ground turkey, stirring until evenly browned and crumbly, about 5 minutes. Season with salt and pepper.

3   In a blender, add the onion, garlic, bell pepper, and tomatoes. Pulse until fully mixed.

4   Stir in the mixture and olives, brine, cumin, and bay leaf, combining well with turkey. Simmer for 12 to 15 minutes.

5   Remove the bay leaf before serving. Top with fresh cilantro if using and serve with brown rice.

anita's tip To add a kick of heat, add a sliced jalapeño or serrano pepper in the blender with the rest of the vegetables. Turkey picadillo is an ideal dish for meal prepping! You can refrigerate the leftovers for up to 4 days or freeze the rest for up to 3 months.

| | S, DF | EASE: ●○○ | MAKES: 1 serving | TIME: 20 minutes |

vietnamese-inspired chicken rolls

what you'll need:

GROUP 1

1 serving = 2 rolls

2 teaspoons (10 ml) extra-virgin olive oil

3¾ ounces (110 g) uncooked chicken breast, skinless and boneless, diced

¼ teaspoon garlic powder

¼ teaspoon onion powder

¼ teaspoon salt

⅛ teaspoon ground black pepper

¾ ounces (25 g) dry cellophane noodles

2 rice paper wrappers

½ cup (70 g) cucumber, peeled and diced

⅓ cup (20 g) bean sprouts

1 tablespoon (15 ml) low-sodium soy sauce

GROUPS 2 & 3

1 serving = 3 rolls

2 teaspoons (10 ml) extra-virgin olive oil

5 ounces (140 g) uncooked chicken breast, skinless and boneless, diced

½ teaspoon garlic powder

½ teaspoon onion powder

¼ teaspoon salt

⅛ teaspoon ground black pepper

1 ounce (30 g) dry cellophane noodles

3 rice paper wrappers

½ cup (70 g) peeled and diced cucumber

⅓ cup (20 g) bean sprouts

1 tablespoon (15 ml) low-sodium soy sauce

1 Heat the oil over medium-high heat in a medium, nonstick skillet. Season the chicken breast with garlic powder, onion powder, salt, and pepper. Brown on the skillet for 3 to 4 minutes on both sides, or until the chicken is cooked through. Remove from the heat.

2 While the chicken is being browned, cook the cellophane noodles according to package instructions. Rinse with cold water for a second or two to chill. Set aside.

3 Fill a large bowl with warm water. Dip each rice paper wrapper into hot water to soften. On a clean work surface, pile each wrapper with the chicken, noodles, cucumber, and sprouts in the center of the rice paper, leaving an empty space around the toppings. Drizzle lightly with soy sauce.

4 Roll up the wrappers up like a burrito: Pull the bottom up and over the center mound. Fold the two sides toward the center. Roll upward until you hit the edge of the rice paper and the chicken roll is tightly sealed. Serve the rolls immediately

anita's tip Not only do these non-fried, fresh spring rolls make one the quickest lunch fixes in the book, they are absolutely delicious. To make this recipe plant-based, try replacing the chicken with crispy tofu.

LUNCH

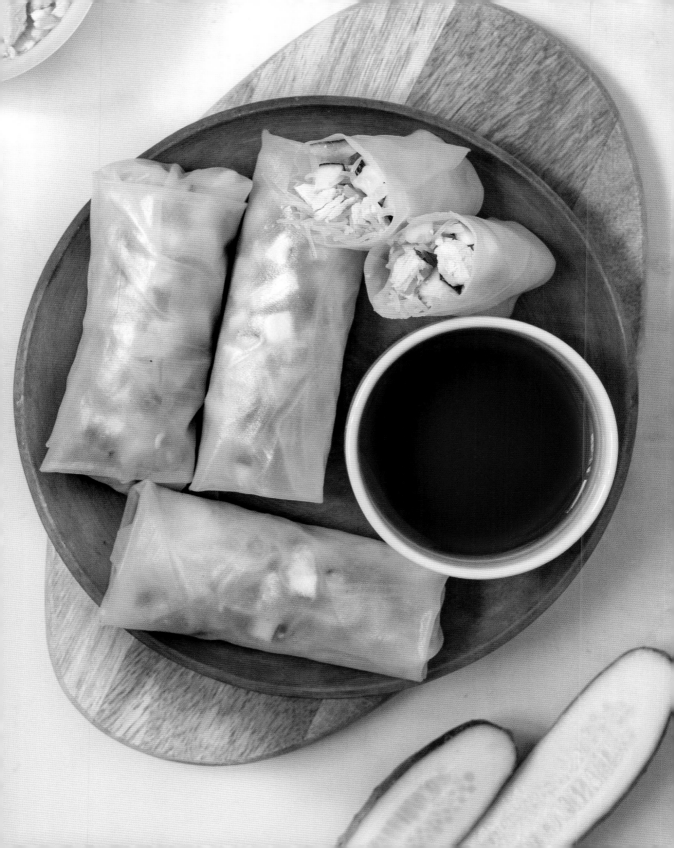

S, DF, GF

 EASE:
●●●

MAKES:
2 servings

 TIME:
30 minutes

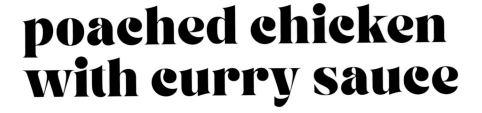

poached chicken with curry sauce

what you'll need:

GROUP 1

3 ounces (85 g) dry brown basmati rice, well rinsed

7½ ounces (215 g) uncooked chicken breast, skinless and boneless

4 quick sprays of cooking oil

2 tablespoons (15 g) thinly sliced yellow onion

2 cloves garlic, finely minced

½ teaspoon curry powder

¼ teaspoon ground ginger

½ tablespoon (4 g) garam masala

Dash of cayenne pepper

½ cup (120 ml) canned full-fat coconut milk, unsweetened

2 teaspoons (10 ml) tamari sauce

½ small cucumber, thinly sliced

1 cup (55 g) roughly chopped lettuce

GROUPS 2 & 3

4 ounces (115 g) dry brown basmati rice, well rinsed

10 ounces (285 g) uncooked chicken breast, skinless and boneless

4 quick sprays of cooking oil

2 tablespoons (15 g) thinly sliced yellow onion

2 cloves garlic, finely minced

2 teaspoons (10 ml) tamari sauce

1 teaspoon curry powder

¼ teaspoon ground ginger

½ tablespoon (4 g) garam masala

Dash of cayenne pepper

½ cup (120 ml) canned full-fat coconut milk, unsweetened

½ small cucumber, thinly sliced

1 cup (55 g) roughly chopped lettuce

1 Prepare the rice according to the package directions. Fluff with a fork and set aside.

2 Fill a pan with water and bring it to a boil. Add the chicken breast, adding more water over the chicken if necessary to ensure it is fully submerged. Poach the chicken for 7 to 8 minutes, until cooked through. Slice.

3 Meanwhile, heat a small non-stick pan over medium heat and lightly coat it with cooking spray. Add the onion. Cook for 2 to 3 minutes. Add the coconut milk and reduce to a simmer. Add the tamari sauce, curry powder, and other spices, if using, stir to combine, and cook for 5 to 6 minutes. Set aside.

4 Add the rice, lettuce, and cucumber to two bowls with the sliced poached chicken. Top with curry sauce.

anita's tip Canned coconut milk is a great base for Asian-inspired sauces: 2 tablespoons (30 ml) count as one portion of fat.

LUNCH

homemade chicken lo mein

what you'll need:

GROUP 1

2 tablespoons (30 ml) low-sodium soy sauce

2 tablespoons (30 g) hoisin sauce

1 teaspoon toasted sesame oil

2½ ounces (70g) dry lo mein egg noodles

1 tablespoon (15 ml) extra-virgin olive oil, divided

7½ ounces (215 g) uncooked chicken breast, skinless and boneless, cut into thin strips

1 medium carrot, grated

⅓ cup (45 g) frozen peas

2 cloves garlic, minced

1 cup (30 g) baby spinach

GROUP 2 & 3

2 tablespoons (30 ml) low-sodium soy sauce

2 tablespoons (30 g) hoisin sauce

1 teaspoon toasted sesame oil

3½ ounces (100 g) dry lo mein egg noodles

1 tablespoon (15 ml) extra-virgin olive oil, divided

10 ounces (285 g) uncooked chicken breast, skinless and boneless, cut into thin strips

1 medium carrot, grated

⅓ cup (45 g) frozen peas

2 cloves garlic, minced

1 cup (30 g) baby spinach

1 In a small bowl, whisk together the soy sauce, hoisin sauce, and sesame oil. Set aside.

2 Bring a medium pot of water to a boil. Add the egg noodles and cook according to package directions. Drain and set aside.

3 In a large, nonstick pan set over medium heat, add ½ tablespoon (8 ml) of olive oil. Add the chicken and cook, stirring frequently, until cooked through. Remove the chicken from the pan and set it aside.

4 Add the remaining olive oil on the pan. Add the carrots and peas to the pan. Cook until the vegetables are tender, about 3 minutes. Add the garlic and cook for 1 minute until fragrant.

5 Add the spinach, cooked noodles, chicken, and prepared sauce to the pan. Cook, stirring, until combined and the spinach is wilted, about 2 minutes.

anita's tip This is the easiest lo mein you will ever make! If you can't find lo mein egg noodles, use regular egg noodles or spaghetti.

tofu veggie stir-fry

what you'll need:

GROUP 1

3 ounces (85 g) dry soba noodles
12 ounces (340 g) firm tofu
1½ tablespoons (12 g) cornstarch, divided
1 teaspoon extra-virgin olive oil
2 tablespoons (30 ml) low-sodium soy sauce
2 teaspoons (10 ml) toasted sesame oil
1 cup (70 g) chopped fresh broccoli florets
1 cup (150 g) chopped red bell peppers
1 cup (70 g) sliced mushrooms
1 cup (100 g) chopped green beans
2 cloves garlic, minced
1 teaspoon fresh ginger, grated
½ cup (65 g) chopped carrots
Extra-virgin olive oil cooking spray, optional
1 tablespoon (8 g) sesame seeds

GROUPS 2 & 3

4 ounces (115 g) dry soba noodles
1 lb. (455 g) firm tofu
1½ tablespoons (12 g) cornstarch, divided
1 teaspoon extra-virgin olive oil
2 tablespoons (30 ml) low-sodium soy sauce
2 teaspoons (10 ml) toasted sesame oil
1 cup (70 g) chopped fresh broccoli florets
1 cup (150 g) chopped red bell peppers
1 cup (70 g) sliced mushrooms
1 cup (100 g) chopped green beans
½ cup (65 g) chopped carrots
2 cloves garlic, minced
1 teaspoon fresh ginger, grated
Extra-virgin olive oil cooking spray, optional
1 tablespoon (8 g) sesame seeds

1 Cook the soba noodles according to package instructions.

2 Remove the tofu from the package and drain out the water. Cut in half lengthwise. Place a towel on top and cover with a heavy object, such as a skillet and allow it to press for 30 minutes.

3 Lightly coat a large, nonstick pan or wok with olive oil over high heat. Sprinkle both sides of tofu lightly with 1 tablespoon (8 g) of cornstarch. Add the tofu and sear until browned, about 3 to 5 minutes per each side. Remove and cut the tofu into small cubes. Set aside.

4 To make the stir-fry sauce, add the soy sauce, sesame oil, 2 tablespoons (30 ml) of water, and the remaining cornstarch in a small bowl. Mix well.

5 In the same pan or wok, add a few extra sprays of cooking oil, if needed. Add the broccoli, bell pepper, and green beans, and cook for 5 minutes. Add the garlic, ginger, and carrot. Drizzle with stir-fry sauce. Toss to coat and stir-fry about 2 to 3 minutes. If the sauce appears too thick, stir in some more water.

6 Add the seared tofu and noodles and stir to coat. Cook until heated through, about 5 minutes on each side. Sprinkle with sesame seeds and serve.

LUNCH

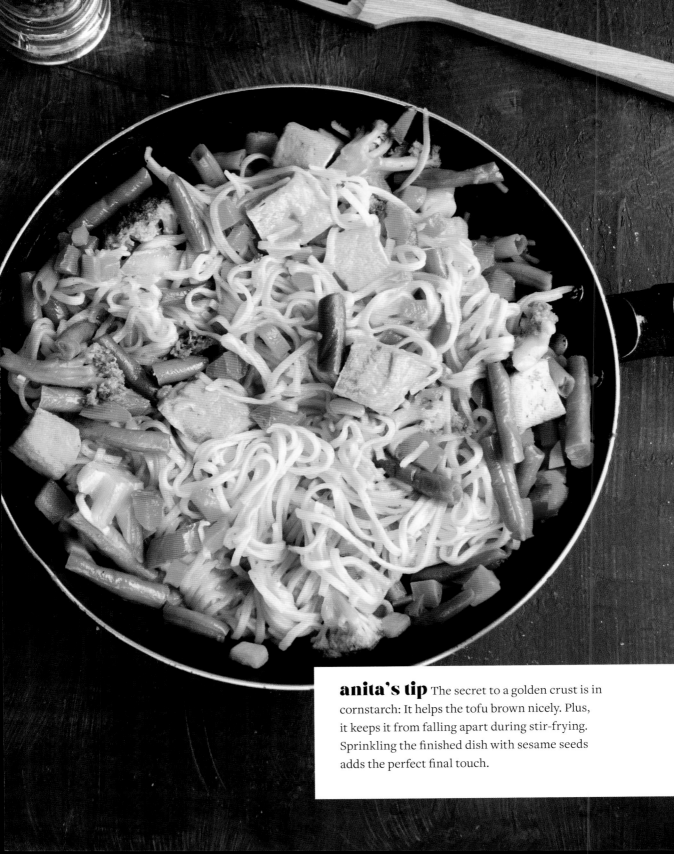

anita's tip The secret to a golden crust is in cornstarch: It helps the tofu brown nicely. Plus, it keeps it from falling apart during stir-frying. Sprinkling the finished dish with sesame seeds adds the perfect final touch.

air-fryer chipotle fish tacos

what you'll need:

GROUP 1
1 serving = 1½ tacos
Fish
¼ cup (35 g) yellow cornmeal
1 teaspoon garlic powder
¼ teaspoon salt
⅛ teaspoon ground black pepper
1 small egg
10 ounces (285 g) uncooked cod filet
Extra-virgin olive oil cooking spray

Chipotle Sauce
⅓ cup (65 g) plain nonfat Greek yogurt
2 tablespoons (30 g) low-fat mayonnaise
1 chipotle pepper in canned adobo sauce, plus sauce to taste
2 teaspoons (10 ml) fresh lime juice

To Serve
3 (4-inch [10-cm]) corn tortillas
⅔ cup (45 g) thinly sliced red cabbage
1 teaspoon fresh lime juice
¼ cup (65 g) pico de gallo
¼ avocado, thinly sliced
1 jalapeño, thinly sliced, optional
Fresh cilantro, thinly sliced

GROUPS 2 & 3
1 serving = 2 tacos
Fish
⅓ cup (45 g) yellow cornmeal
1 teaspoon garlic powder
¼ teaspoon salt
⅛ teaspoon ground black pepper
1 small egg
12½ ounces (355 g) uncooked cod filet
Extra-virgin olive oil cooking spray

Chipotle Sauce
⅔ cup (135 g) plain nonfat Greek yogurt
2 tablespoons (30 g) low-fat mayonnaise
1 tablespoon (15 ml) fresh lime juice
1 chipotle pepper in canned adobo sauce, plus sauce to taste

To Serve
4 (4-inch [10-cm]) corn tortillas
⅔ cup (45 g) thinly sliced red cabbage
1 teaspoon fresh lime juice
¼ avocado, thinly sliced
¼ cup (65 g) pico de gallo
1 jalapeño, thinly sliced, optional
Fresh cilantro, thinly sliced

1   To make the fish, place two small bowls on the counter. In the first bowl, whisk together the cornmeal, garlic powder, salt, and pepper. In the second bowl, beat the egg.

2   Cut the cod into long strips. One by one, dip each side of cod strips lightly in the seasoned cornmeal mix, then the egg, then again lightly in cornmeal.

3   Preheat the air fryer to 400°F (200°C). Coat the air-fryer basket with cooking spray. Arrange the coated fish pieces in the basket spaced apart. Coat thoroughly with cooking spray. Cook in the air fryer until the fish is lightly browned and flakes easily, about 10 to 12 minutes. Remove from the air fryer and set aside.

4   Place the corn tortillas inside two pieces of aluminum foil and mold into a U-shaped

LUNCH

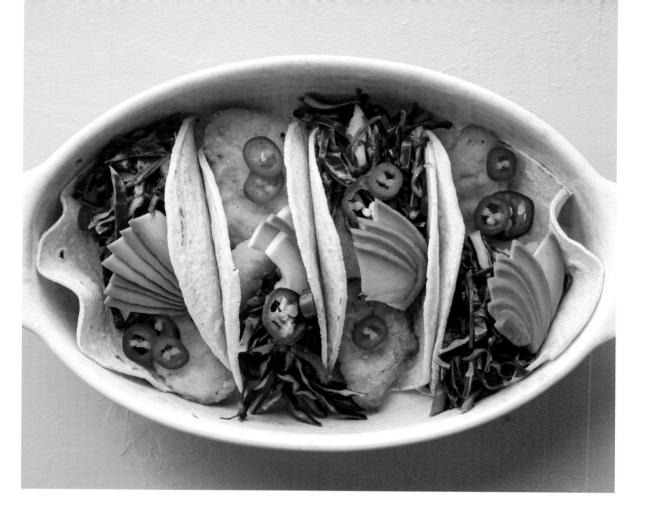

taco form. Place in the air fryer and heat until the tortillas have reached desired firmness.

5 To make the chipotle sauce, combine the yogurt, mayonnaise, chipotle pepper, and 2 teaspoons (10 ml) lime juice in a blender. Blend until smooth. Taste and add adobo sauce from the chipotle can for added spiciness, if desired.

6 Spread the chipotle sauce on the tortillas. Divide the fish and cabbage among the tortillas and lightly drizzle with 1 teaspoon of lime juice. Add sliced avocado, 1 tablespoon (15 g) of pico de gallo, and jalapeño (if using) on each tortilla. Top generously with leftover chipotle sauce and fresh cilantro.

anita's tip Air-fried tacos are the perfect alternative for those crunchy, rustic taco truck–style tacos that are full of flavor. You can use any lean, non-oily white fish filets, such as cod, sea bass, or mahi-mahi. Refer to the swap table (page 64) for the right replacement amounts.

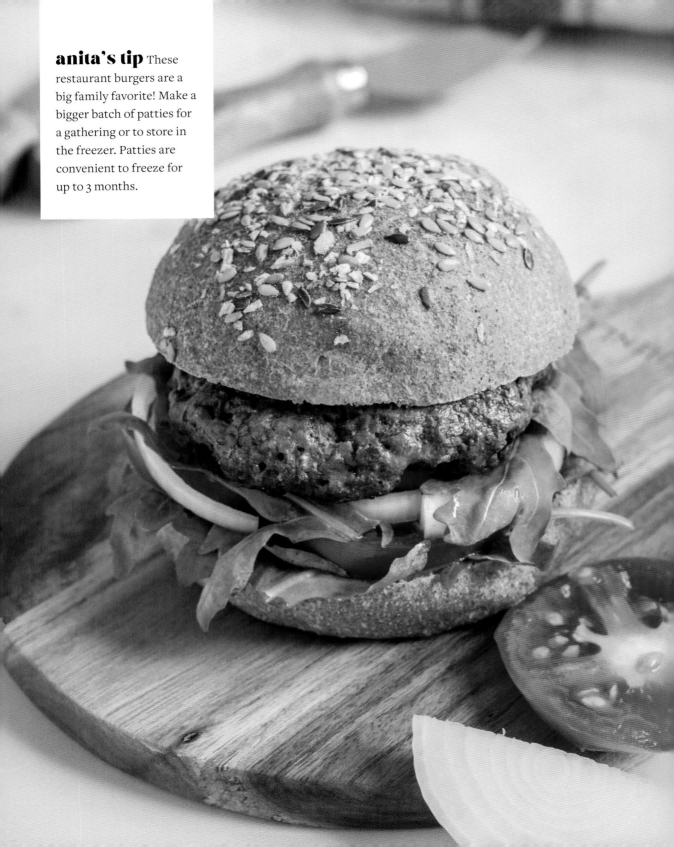

anita's tip These restaurant burgers are a big family favorite! Make a bigger batch of patties for a gathering or to store in the freezer. Patties are convenient to freeze for up to 3 months.

| | S, GF | EASE: ●○○ | MAKES: 1 serving | TIME: 20 minutes |

restaurant-style all-american burger

what you'll need:

GROUP 1
Burger
3 ¾ ounces (110 g) uncooked lean ground beef, 95%
1 teaspoon finely chopped yellow onion
1 teaspoon Worcestershire sauce
½ teaspoon liquid smoke
1 teaspoon Dijon mustard
3 rings red onion
¼ cup (45 g) sliced fresh tomato
¼ cup (15 g) shredded lettuce
1 tablespoon (15 g) shredded cheddar cheese
Extra-virgin olive oil cooking spray
1 burger bun of choice
Pickles, optional

Sauce
1 tablespoon (15 g) low-fat mayonnaise
1 tablespoon (15 g) ketchup, no added sugar

GROUPS 2 & 3
Burger
5 ounces (140 g) uncooked lean ground beef, 95%
1 teaspoon finely chopped yellow onion
1 teaspoon Worcestershire sauce
½ teaspoon liquid smoke
1 teaspoon Dijon mustard
3 rings red onion
¼ cup (45 g) sliced fresh tomato
¼ cup (15 g) shredded lettuce
1 tablespoon (15 g) shredded cheddar cheese
Extra-virgin olive oil cooking spray
1 burger bun of choice
Pickles, optional

Sauce
1 tablespoon (15 g) low-fat mayonnaise
1 tablespoon (15 g) ketchup, no added sugar

1   To make the patty, add the ground beef, onion, Worcestershire sauce, liquid smoke, and Dijon mustard to a large bowl. Without overworking the meat, mix with your hands until evenly combined. Shape into a patty.

2   Place the patty on a preheated grill or grill pan over medium-high heat. Cook 3 minutes on one side, flip and top with the cheese, then cook for 3 minutes, or until cooked through and the cheese is melted. Note: You won't need any oil for cooking given the fat concentration of ground beef.

3   Meanwhile, make a burger sauce by combining mayonnaise and ketchup in a small bowl.

4   Spray each side of the burger bun with 2 quick sprays of cooking oil, then place on the grill or grill pan until warm and lightly toasted.

5   Serve the patty on a toasted burger bun with lettuce, tomatoes, onion, burger sauce, and pickles, if using.

GROUP 1: *This recipe contains one burger bun, which counts as two portions of starch. It requires borrowing ½ portion of starch from breakfast, AM snack, or dinner.*

LUNCH

korean-style spicy garlic shrimp pasta

what you'll need:

GROUP 1

3 ounces (85 g) dry spaghetti of choice

15 ounces (425 g) raw jumbo shrimp, peeled and deveined

1 tablespoon (8 g) cornstarch

1 tablespoon (15 ml) low-sodium soy sauce

1 tablespoon (8 ml) fish sauce

2 teaspoons (15 g) honey

1 tablespoon (8 g) Korean gochugaru chili powder

1 tablespoon extra-virgin olive oil

1 tablespoon (15 g) unsalted butter

2 cloves garlic, minced

1 scallion, sliced

GROUPS 2 & 3

4 ounces (115 g) dry spaghetti of choice

1¼ lb. (565 g) raw jumbo shrimp, peeled and deveined

1 tablespoon (8 g) cornstarch

1 tablespoon (15 ml) low-sodium soy sauce

½ tablespoon (8 ml) fish sauce

2 teaspoons (15 g) honey

1 tablespoon (8 g) Korean gochugaru chili powder

1 tablespoon extra-virgin olive oil

1 tablespoon (15 g) unsalted butter

2 cloves garlic, minced

1 scallion, sliced

1 In a large pot, bring water to a boil. Cook the pasta according to package directions until al dente. Drain the pasta and set aside.

2 Meanwhile, combine the shrimp and cornstarch in a mixing bowl and set it aside. In a second bowl, combine the soy sauce, fish sauce, honey, and gochugaru with 1 tablespoon (15 ml) of water. Mix well.

3 Heat the oil in a large, nonstick skillet over high heat. Add the shrimp and sear evenly, no more than 2 to 3 minutes per side. Add the butter and garlic and cook for 1 minute. Pour the sauce mixture on top and toss the shrimp to coat.

4 Add the cooked pasta to the skillet with the scallions and toss to combine.

anita's tip Korean gochugaru has a unique smoky and slightly sweet flavor that makes the taste different from regular chili powder. To turn up the heat, you can add more gochugaru powder to taste in step 2.

LUNCH

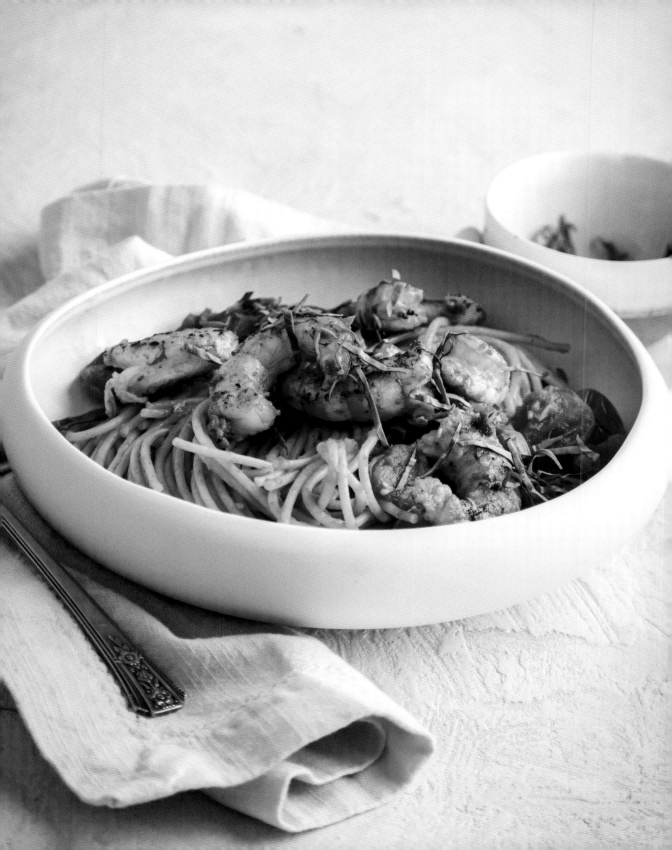

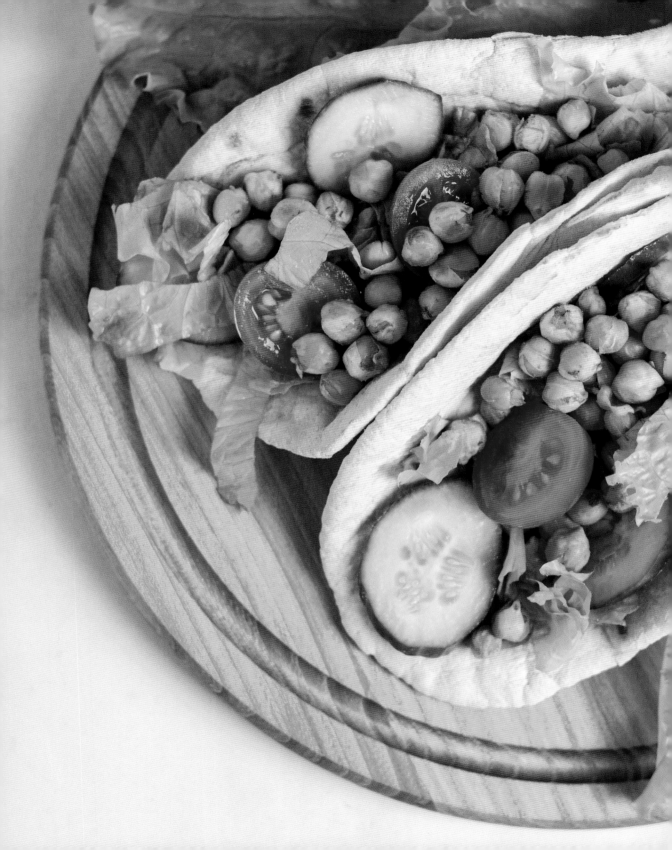

S, V

EASE:
●●○

MAKES:
2 servings

TIME:
45 minutes

buffalo roasted chickpea wraps

what you'll need:

GROUP 1

1 serving = 1½ wraps

1 cup (240 g) canned chickpeas, rinsed and well-drained

2 teaspoons (10 ml) extra-virgin olive oil

¼ cup (60 ml) Buffalo hot sauce, divided, more to taste

3 (4-inch [10-cm]) flour pita breads

½ cup (30 g) shredded lettuce

½ cup (75 g) cherry tomatoes, halved

½ small cucumber, thinly sliced

⅔ cup (160 ml) Better Than Store-Bought Ranch Sauce (page 192)

GROUPS 2 & 3

1 serving = 2 wraps

1½ cups (360 g) canned chickpeas, rinsed and well-drained

2 teaspoons (10 ml) extra-virgin olive oil

¼ cup (60 ml) Buffalo hot sauce, divided, more to taste

4 (4-inch [10-cm]) flour pita breads

½ cup (30 g) shredded lettuce

½ cup (75 g) cherry tomatoes, halved

½ small cucumber, thinly sliced

⅔ cup (160 ml) Better Than Store-Bought Ranch Sauce (page 192)

1 Preheat the oven to 400°F (200°C). Pat the chickpeas dry and place them in a small mixing bowl. Toss them lightly with oil. Place in a baking dish.

2 Roast the chickpeas until golden brown and crispy, 30 to 35 minutes. Remove them from the oven and coat with 2 tablespoons (30 ml) of Buffalo hot sauce. Return to the oven until the hot sauce has dried, about 3 to 5 minutes. Remove from the oven, and coat again with 1 tablespoon (15 ml) of hot sauce. Return to the oven and bake for 3 to 5 minutes.

3 Divide the roasted chickpeas, lettuce, tomatoes, and cucumber evenly among the pita breads. Drizzle with the remaining hot sauce. Serve with ranch sauce as a dip, or drizzle on the pita wraps with more hot sauce, if desired.

GF: *To make this recipe gluten-free, choose a gluten-free pita brand.*

anita's tip Roasted chickpeas make the perfect crunchy snack, too—rich in both protein and carbs. A 1/4 cup (60 g) serving counts as a portion of protein, and 1/2 cup (120 g) as a portion of starch!

argentinian-style steak with chimichurri

what you'll need:

GROUP 1

2 cloves garlic, finely minced

1 teaspoon onion powder

1 teaspoon salt

¼ teaspoon ground black pepper

1 tablespoon (15 ml) fresh lime juice

2 teaspoons (10 ml) extra-virgin olive oil

4 quick sprays cooking spray

15 ounces (425 g) uncooked flank steak, or other lean cut of beef

2 tablespoons (30 ml) Mabel's Chimichurri Criollo sauce (page 190)

GROUP 2

2 cloves garlic, finely minced

1 teaspoon onion powder

1 teaspoon salt

¼ teaspoon ground black pepper

1 tablespoon (15 ml) fresh lime juice

2 tablespoons (30 ml) extra-virgin olive oil, divided

15 ounces (425 g) uncooked flank steak, or other lean cut of beef

2 tablespoons (30 ml) Mabel's Chimichurri Criollo sauce (page 190)

GROUP 3

2 cloves garlic, finely minced

1 teaspoon onion powder

1 teaspoon salt

¼ teaspoon ground black pepper

1 tablespoon (15 ml) fresh lime juice

8 teaspoons (40 ml) extra-virgin olive oil, divided

1¼ lb. (565 g) uncooked flank steak, or other lean cut of beef

¼ cup (60 ml) Mabel's Chimichurri Criollo sauce (page 190)

1   Make a marinade by mixing the garlic, onion powder, salt, pepper, lime juice, and 2 teaspoons (10 ml) of oil (group 1), or 1 tablespoon (15 ml) of oil (groups 2 and 3). Combine with the uncooked steak and place it in a large zip-top bag. Let marinate for at least 1 hour or overnight.

2   Preheat a grill or large grill pan over medium-high heat and coat with 4 quick sprays of cooking spray, or the remaining olive oil as indicated for your group. Sear the steak for 6 to 8 minutes on each side, until heavily browned on the outside and slightly pink in the middle for medium-well. If you want it well-done, lower the heat and cook for 2 to 3 minutes. Avoid overcooking so the steak doesn't become dry.

3   Let it rest on a plastic cutting board for 5 minutes. Thinly slice the steak across the grain and serve with chimichurri sauce on top. Serve with a side of your choice (1 portion starch per serving), and grilled vegetables or a green salad on the side.

DINNER

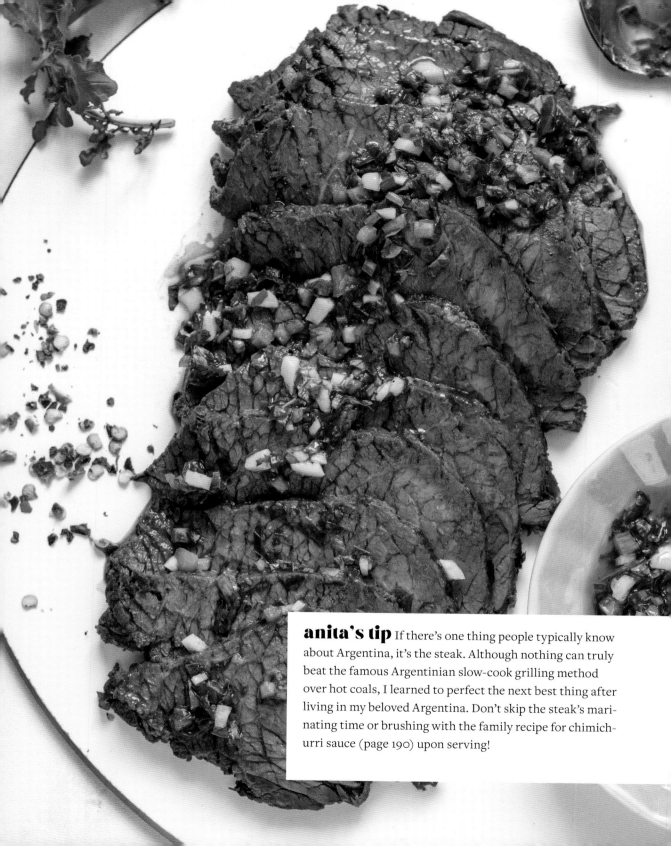

anita's tip If there's one thing people typically know about Argentina, it's the steak. Although nothing can truly beat the famous Argentinian slow-cook grilling method over hot coals, I learned to perfect the next best thing after living in my beloved Argentina. Don't skip the steak's marinating time or brushing with the family recipe for chimichurri sauce (page 190) upon serving!

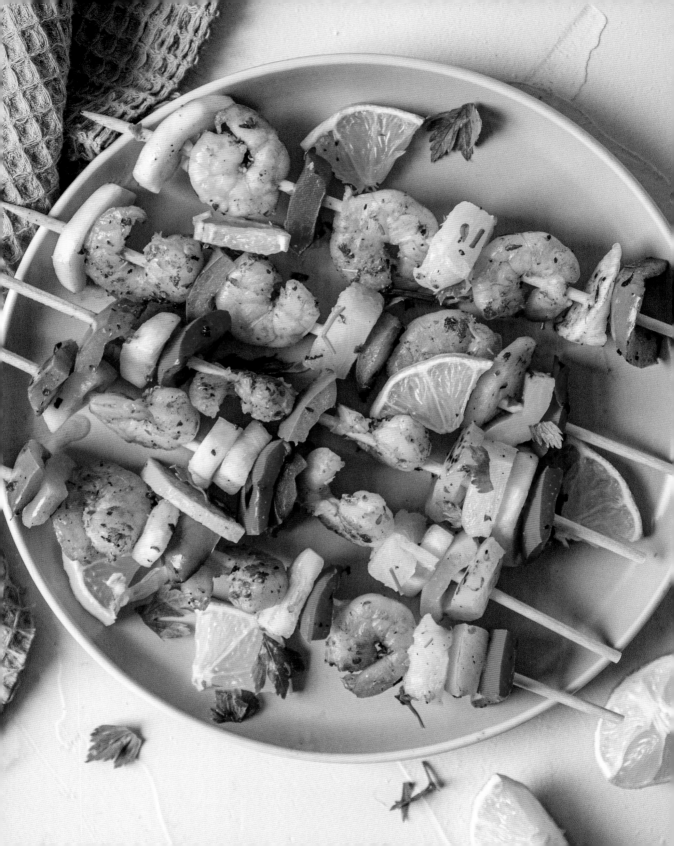

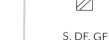

| S, DF, GF | EASE: ●○○ | MAKES: 2 servings | TIME: 25 minutes |

jumbo shrimp skewers

what you'll need:

GROUP 1

2 teaspoons (10 ml) extra-virgin olive oil

½ tablespoon (8 ml) fresh lemon juice

½ teaspoon dried parsley

½ teaspoon smoked paprika

½ teaspoon garlic powder

¼ teaspoon salt

¼ teaspoon ground black pepper

15 ounces (425 g) raw jumbo shrimp, peeled and deveined

1 medium zucchini, cut into chunks

1 red bell pepper, cut into pieces

1 green bell pepper, cut into pieces

GROUP 2

4 teaspoons (20 ml) extra-virgin olive oil

½ tablespoon (8 ml) fresh lemon juice

½ teaspoon dried parsley

½ teaspoon smoked paprika

½ teaspoon garlic powder

¼ teaspoon salt

¼ teaspoon ground black pepper

15 ounces (425 g) raw jumbo shrimp, peeled and deveined

1 medium zucchini, cut into chunks

1 red bell pepper, cut into pieces
1 green bell pepper, cut into pieces

GROUP 3

2 tablespoons (30 ml) extra-virgin olive oil

½ tablespoon (8 ml) fresh lemon juice

½ teaspoon dried parsley

½ teaspoon smoked paprika

½ teaspoon garlic powder

¼ teaspoon salt

¼ teaspoon ground black pepper

1¼ lb. (565 g) raw jumbo shrimp, peeled and deveined

1 medium zucchini, cut into chunks

1 red bell pepper, cut into pieces

1 green bell pepper, cut into pieces

1 Combine the oil, lemon juice, parsley, smoked paprika, garlic powder, salt, and pepper in a large bowl. Mix well. Add the shrimp to the bowl and toss to coat. Marinate for at least 15 minutes.

2 Slide the shrimp and veggies on skewers in an alternating order.

3 Preheat a grill or large, nonstick skillet over medium-high heat and coat with cooking spray. Cook for 2 to 3 minutes on each side until the color of shrimp is pink and opaque.

4 Serve with a side of your choice (1 portion starch per serving).

anita's tip These skewers are equally delicious with scallops, seitan cubes, tofu, or cubed chicken breast. If using wooden skewers, make sure you soak them in water for 30 minutes. Otherwise, they'll cook with the food when you place them on the grill.

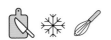   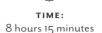

| | S, DF | EASE: ●●○ | MAKES: 4 servings | TIME: 8 hours 15 minutes |

slow-cooker pork ramen soup

what you'll need:

GROUP 1

1 tablespoon (15 ml) extra-virgin olive oil

10 ounces (285 g) uncooked lean pork tenderloin, trimmed and sliced

1 cup (70 g) sliced carrots

1 cup (100 g) sliced scallions, plus ½ cup more for garnish

1 teaspoon fresh ginger, peeled and finely chopped

4 cloves garlic, chopped

4 cups (940 ml) low-sodium chicken broth

2 tablespoons (30 ml) low-sodium soy sauce

4 ounces (115 g) dry ramen noodles

4 small eggs

1 tablespoon (8 g) sesame seeds

GROUP 2

4 teaspoons (20 ml) extra-virgin olive oil

10 ounces (285 g) uncooked lean pork tenderloin, trimmed and sliced

1 cup (70 g) sliced carrots

1 cup (100 g) sliced scallions, plus ½ cup more for garnish

1 teaspoon fresh ginger, peeled and finely chopped

6 cloves garlic, chopped

4 cups (940 ml) low-sodium chicken broth

3 tablespoons (45 ml) low-sodium soy sauce

4 ounces (115 g) dry ramen noodles

4 small eggs

¼ cup (30 g) sesame seeds

GROUP 3

8 teaspoons (40 ml) extra-virgin olive oil

15 ounces (425 g) uncooked lean pork tenderloin, trimmed and sliced

1 cup (70 g) sliced carrots

1 cup (100 g) sliced scallions, plus ½ cup more for garnish

1 teaspoon fresh ginger, peeled and finely chopped

4 cloves garlic, chopped

4 cups (940 ml) low-sodium chicken broth

2 tablespoons (30 ml) low-sodium soy sauce

4 ounces (115 g) dry ramen noodles

4 small eggs

¼ cup (35 g) sesame seeds

1 In a large, nonstick skillet, heat the oil over medium-high heat until hot. Add the pork, in multiple batches if needed, and cook 3 to 4 minutes per side until browned. Transfer the pork to a slow cooker.

2 Pour in the vegetables, broth, and soy sauce. Cover and cook on low for 6 to 8 hours, or until the pork is tender. Using a spoon, skim off and discard any fat from the surface of the broth.

3 Cook the ramen noodles as directed on the package and drain.

4 Meanwhile, bring a small pot of water to a simmer. Add the eggs and cook for 6 minutes. Adjust the heat to keep a consistent temperature. Remove the eggs from the water and run them under cold water until cool. Peel and slice the soft-boiled eggs in half.

DINNER

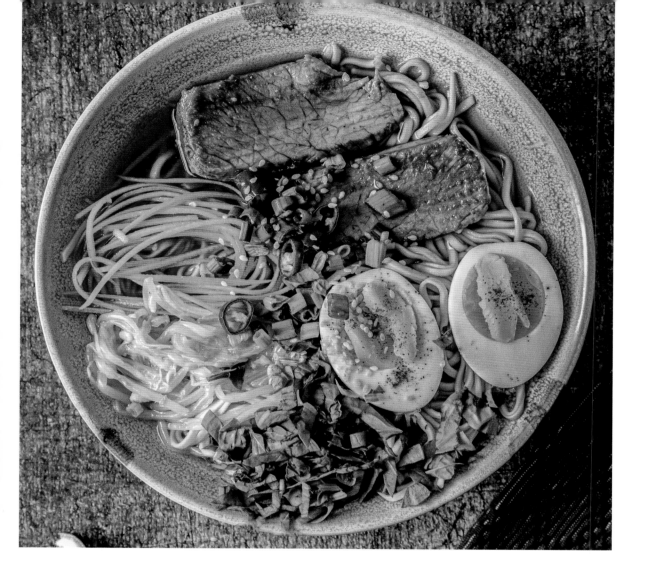

5 To serve, divide the noodles evenly among individual bowls. Ladle the broth and pork over the noodles, dividing evenly. Add two egg halves in each bowl. Top with sesame seeds evenly on each bowl. Serve with extra scallions.

anita's tip A slow cooker is your BFF when it comes to making hearty meals like this one. With a little work before and after you load in the ingredients, letting the slow cooker do the rest almost feels like cheating! You can make chicken ramen the same way by swapping sliced pork with sliced chicken breast.

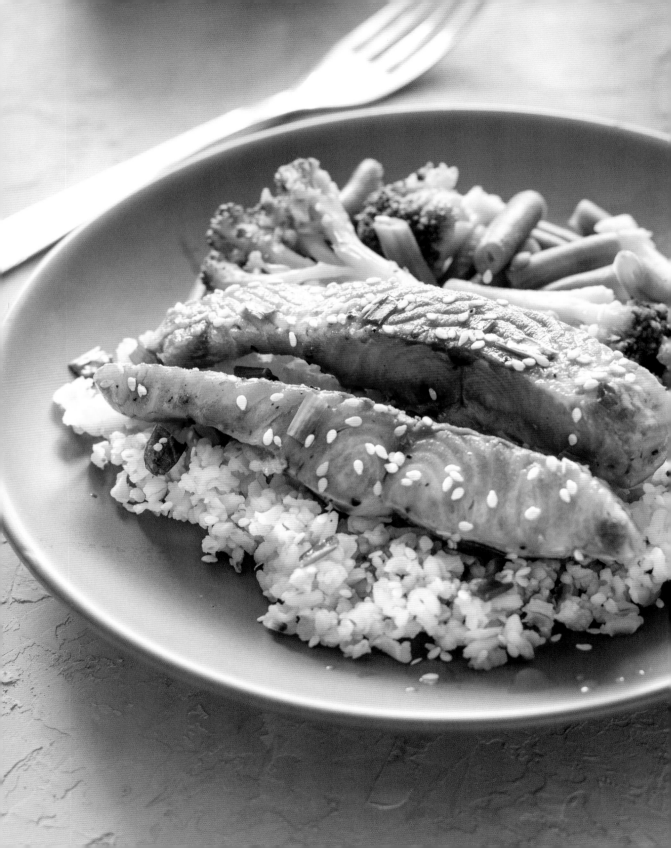

baked teriyaki sesame salmon

what you'll need:

GROUP 1

1 ounce (30 g) dry brown rice, well rinsed
3¾ ounces (110 g) uncooked salmon filet
1½ tablespoons (25 ml) teriyaki sauce, divided
1 teaspoon fresh ginger, minced
1 clove garlic, minced
4 quick sprays of cooking oil
1 cup (100 g) trimmed green beans
1 cup (90 g) broccoli florets
1 tablespoon (8 g) sesame seeds
1 tablespoon (6 g) finely sliced scallions

GROUP 2

1 ounce (30 g) dry brown rice, well rinsed
3¾ ounces (110 g) uncooked salmon filet
1½ tablespoons (25 ml) teriyaki sauce, divided
1 teaspoon fresh ginger, minced
1 clove garlic, minced
1 teaspoon extra-virgin olive oil
1 cup (100 g) trimmed green beans
1 cup (90 g) broccoli florets

1 tablespoon (8 g) sesame seeds
1 tablespoon (6 g) finely sliced scallions

GROUP 3

1 ounce (30 g) dry brown rice, well rinsed
5 ounces (140 g) uncooked salmon filet
1½ tablespoons (25 ml) teriyaki sauce, divided
1 teaspoon fresh ginger, minced
1 clove garlic, minced
2 teaspoons (10 ml) extra-virgin olive oil
1 cup (100 g) trimmed green beans
1 cup (90 g) broccoli florets
1 tablespoon (8 g) sesame seeds
1 tablespoon (6 g) finely sliced scallions

anita's tip This recipe uses store-bought teriyaki sauce to save time, but you can make it at home, too! You'll find the recipe on the website.

1 Make the rice according to the package directions. In the last 10 minutes, place a steamer insert above the pot to steam green beans and broccoli.

2 In a medium bowl, combine 1 tablespoon (15 ml) of teriyaki sauce, ginger, and garlic. Add salmon, turn to coat, and let marinate for 10 minutes.

3 Preheat the oven to 450°F (230°C). Coat a small baking sheet lightly with oil. Bake for about 12 to 15 minutes, or until the salmon is cooked through.

4 Spoon the rice onto a plate, then add the salmon and vegetables. Drizzle the salmon with the remaining teriyaki sauce. Sprinkle with sesame seeds and scallions.

spicy turkey chili

what you'll need:

GROUP 1

1 teaspoon extra-virgin olive oil

7½ ounces (215 g) uncooked ground turkey breast, 93–99% lean

½ cup (80 g) chopped yellow onion

2 cloves garlic, minced

½ red bell pepper, chopped

¼ cup (25 g) chopped celery

2 large serrano peppers, diced, plus more to taste

½ teaspoon dried oregano

1 teaspoon chili powder, or more to taste

¼ teaspoon ground cumin

½ cup (90 g) canned diced tomatoes, fire-roasted or regular

½ cup (120 ml) low-sodium chicken broth

½ teaspoon salt

¼ teaspoon ground black pepper

¾ cup (190 g) canned red kidney beans, drained

⅓ cup (55 g) corn, drained

2 tablespoons (15 g) shredded cheddar cheese

GROUP 2

1 tablespoon (15 ml) extra-virgin olive oil

7½ ounces (215 g) uncooked ground turkey breast, 93–99% lean

½ cup (80 g) chopped yellow onion

2 cloves garlic, minced

½ red bell pepper, chopped

¼ cup (25 g) chopped celery

2 large serrano peppers, diced, plus more to taste

½ teaspoon dried oregano

1 teaspoon chili powder, or more to taste

¼ teaspoon ground cumin

½ cup (90 g) canned diced tomatoes, fire-roasted or regular

½ cup (120 ml) low-sodium chicken broth

½ teaspoon salt

¼ teaspoon ground black pepper

¾ cup (190 g) canned red kidney beans, drained

⅓ cup (55 g) corn, drained

2 tablespoons (15 g) shredded cheddar cheese

GROUP 3

4 teaspoons (20 ml) extra-virgin olive oil

10 ounces (285 g) uncooked ground turkey breast, 93–99% lean

½ cup (80 g) chopped yellow onion

2 cloves garlic, minced

½ red bell pepper, chopped

¼ cup (25 g) chopped celery

2 large serrano peppers, diced, plus more to taste

½ teaspoon dried oregano

1 teaspoon chili powder, or more to taste

¼ teaspoon ground cumin

½ cup (90 g) canned diced tomatoes, fire-roasted or regular

½ cup (120 ml) low-sodium chicken broth

½ teaspoon salt

¼ teaspoon ground black pepper

¾ cup (190 g) canned red kidney beans, drained

⅓ cup (55 g) corn, drained

¼ cup (30 g) shredded cheddar cheese

1 Heat the oil over high heat in a large heavy pot and add the ground turkey. Cook until the turkey is lightly browned and crumbling, about 5 minutes.

2 Add the onion, garlic, bell pepper, celery, serrano peppers, oregano, chili powder, and cumin. Mix well. Cook for 5 minutes, stirring frequently.

 DINNER

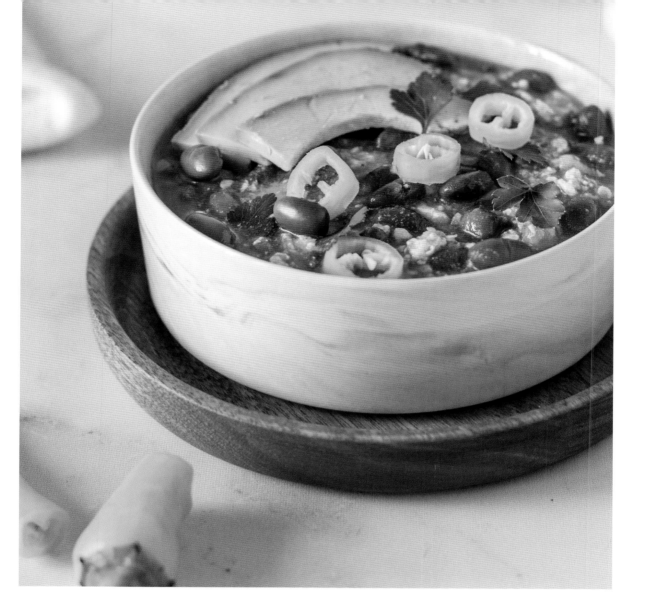

3 Add the tomatoes, chicken broth, salt, and pepper. Bring to a boil, reduce the heat and simmer, stirring occasionally, for 15 minutes.

4 Add the beans and corn. Cook, stirring occasionally, for 10 minutes. Serve in bowls and top with shredded cheddar cheese.

anita's tip You can adjust the heat by substituting serrano for a hotter pepper (see page 80 for a pepper heat chart). Or, if you don't like it too spicy, you can turn it down by swapping for milder peppers, such as jalapeño, poblano, cubanelle, or banana peppers.

S, GF

EASE:
●●○

MAKES:
2 servings

TIME:
25 minutes

loaded taco sweet potatoes

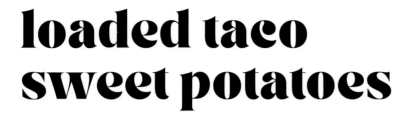

what you'll need:

GROUP 1

2 small (4-ounce [115 g]) sweet potatoes

7½ ounces (215 g) uncooked ground beef, 95% lean

2 teaspoons (5 g) smoked paprika

½ teaspoon garlic powder

½ teaspoon onion powder

½ teaspoon ground cumin

¼ teaspoon chili powder, or more to taste

¼ teaspoon salt

⅛ teaspoon ground black pepper

2 tablespoons (15 g) finely diced onion

2 tablespoons (30 g) tomato paste

2 tablespoons (15 g) shredded cheddar cheese

¼ cup (65 g) pico de gallo

¼ small avocado, diced

Fresh cilantro, chopped

GROUP 2

2 small (4-ounce [115 g]) sweet potatoes

7½ ounces (215 g) uncooked ground beef, 95% lean

2 teaspoons (5 g) smoked paprika

½ teaspoon garlic powder

½ teaspoon onion powder

½ teaspoon ground cumin

¼ teaspoon chili powder, or more to taste

¼ teaspoon salt

⅛ teaspoon ground black pepper

2 tablespoons (15 g) finely diced onion

2 tablespoons (30 g) tomato paste

¼ cup (30 g) shredded cheddar cheese

¼ cup (65 g) pico de gallo

½ small avocado, diced

Fresh cilantro, chopped

GROUP 3

2 small (4-ounce [115 g]) sweet potatoes

10 ounces (285 g) uncooked ground beef, 95% lean

1 tablespoon (7 g) smoked paprika

¾ teaspoon garlic powder

¾ teaspoon onion powder

½ teaspoon ground cumin

¼ teaspoon chili powder, or more to taste

¼ teaspoon salt

⅛ teaspoon ground black pepper

2 tablespoons (15 g) finely diced onion

2 tablespoons (30 g) tomato paste

½ cup (60 g) shredded cheddar cheese

¼ cup (65 g) pico de gallo

½ small avocado, diced

Fresh cilantro, chopped

1 Using a fork, prick a few holes in the sweet potato. Place on a microwave-safe plate and cook on high until tender, about 5 to 6 minutes.

2 Heat a medium, nonstick skillet over medium-high heat. Add the ground beef and smoked paprika, garlic powder, onion powder, cumin, chili powder, salt, and pepper. Cook the beef, breaking up the meat with a spoon, until it's cooked through, about 5 minutes. Reduce the heat to low, add the onion. Cook until the onion is translucent, about 1 to 2 minutes.

3 Whisk 2 tablespoons (30 ml) of water and tomato paste in a measuring cup. Add it to the pan with the meat mixture and stir to coat.

4 To assemble the sweet potato, cut it down the center lengthwise. Lightly mash the flesh

DINNER

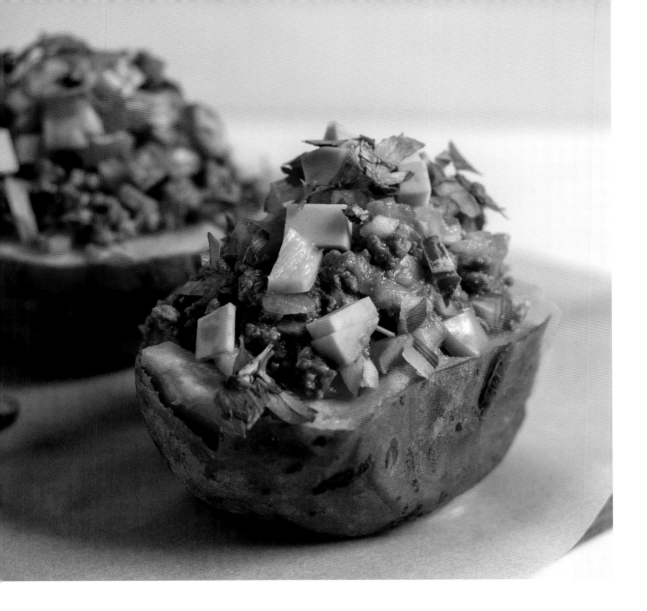

of the potato with a fork and fill each half with taco meat and top with shredded cheese, pico de gallo, avocado, and cilantro.

anita's tip Your family will love these taco-stuffed sweet potatoes! You can use the same base for tacos by simply replacing sweet potatoes with tortillas. If you are meal prepping this recipe, store the toppings and sweet potato separately, and combine upon serving.

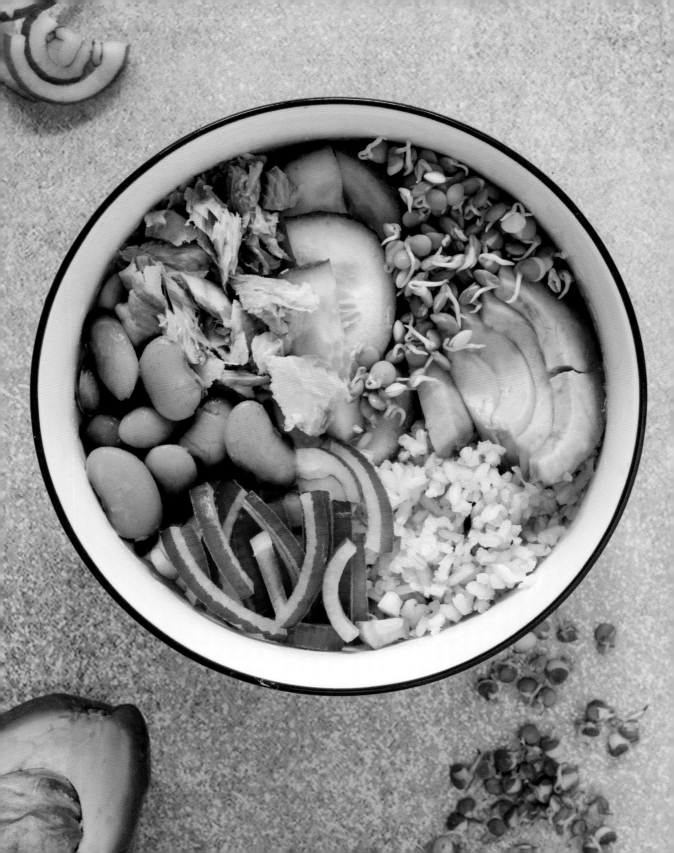

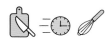

 S, DF, GF

EASE: ●○○

MAKES: 1 serving

TIME: 10 minutes

10-minute tuna bowl

what you'll need:

GROUP 1

¼ cup (40 g) shelled raw edamame
Dash of salt
2 ounces (60 g) tuna in oil, drained
¼ cup (30 g) sliced cucumber
¼ cup (25 g) mung bean sprouts
¼ small avocado, sliced
½ cup (80 g) cooked brown rice
¼ cup (30 g) sliced red onion

GROUP 2

¼ cup (40 g) shelled raw edamame
Dash of salt
2 ounces (60 g) tuna in oil, drained
¼ cup (30 g) sliced cucumber
¼ cup (25 g) mung bean sprouts
½ small avocado, sliced
½ cup (80 g) cooked brown rice
¼ cup (30 g) sliced red onion

GROUP 3

¼ (40 g) raw edamame, shelled
Dash of salt
3 ounces (85 g) tuna in oil, drained
¼ cup (30 g) sliced cucumber
¼ cup (25 g) mung bean sprouts
¾ small avocado, sliced
½ cup (80 g) cooked brown rice
¼ cup (30 g) sliced red onion

1   In a microwave-safe bowl, cover edamame with ¼ cup (60 ml) of water. Microwave on high power for 4 to 6 minutes. Drain any excess water and season with a dash of salt.

2   In a serving bowl, place the edamame, tuna, cucumber, bean sprouts, avocado, cooked brown rice, and red onion in their own sections.

anita's tip Bowls are so easy to put together, especially when you have all the ingredients pre-prepped and ready to go. Swap tuna for chicken, steak, tofu, or slow-cooked barbacoa beef (page 172).

spicy pumpkin chicken soup

what you'll need:

GROUP 1

2 teaspoons (10 ml) extra-virgin olive oil

6 ¼ ounces (175 g) uncooked chicken breast, skinless and boneless, sliced

½ medium yellow onion, finely chopped

1 medium stalk celery, chopped

1 medium carrot, finely chopped

2 large serrano peppers, diced, plus more to taste

2 cloves garlic, minced

4 cups (940 ml) low-sodium or unsalted chicken broth

1 cup (245 g) canned pure pumpkin purée

1 ounce (30 g) dry rice of choice, well rinsed

¼ cup (45 g) canned black beans, drained and rinsed

½ teaspoon ground cumin

½ teaspoon chili powder, or more to taste

½ teaspoon salt

¼ teaspoon ground black pepper

2 small pumpkins, hollowed out, optional

2 tablespoons (8 g) finely chopped fresh parsley

GROUP 2

4 teaspoons (20 ml) extra-virgin olive oil

6 ¼ ounces (175 g) uncooked chicken breast, skinless and boneless

½ medium yellow onion, finely chopped

1 medium stalk celery, chopped

1 medium carrot, finely chopped

2 large serrano peppers, diced, plus more to taste

2 cloves garlic, minced

4 cups (940 ml) low-sodium chicken broth

1 cup (245 g) canned pure pumpkin purée

1 ounce (30 g) dry rice of choice, well rinsed

¼ cup (45 g) canned black beans, drained and rinsed

½ teaspoon ground cumin

½ teaspoon chili powder, or more to taste

½ teaspoon salt

¼ teaspoon ground black pepper

2 small pumpkins, hollowed out, optional

2 tablespoons (8 g) finely chopped fresh parsley

GROUP 3

2 tablespoons (30 ml) extra-virgin olive oil

8 ¾ ounces (250 g) uncooked chicken breast, skinless and boneless, diced

½ medium yellow onion, finely chopped

1 medium stalk celery, chopped

1 medium carrot, finely chopped

2 large serrano peppers, diced, plus more to taste

2 cloves garlic, minced

4 cups (940 ml) low-sodium chicken broth

1 cup (245 g) canned pure pumpkin purée

1 ounce (30 g) dry rice of choice, well rinsed

¼ cup (45 g) canned black beans, drained and rinsed

½ teaspoon ground cumin

½ teaspoon chili powder, or more to taste

½ teaspoon salt

¼ teaspoon ground black pepper

2 small pumpkins, hollowed out, optional

2 tablespoons (8 g) finely chopped fresh parsley

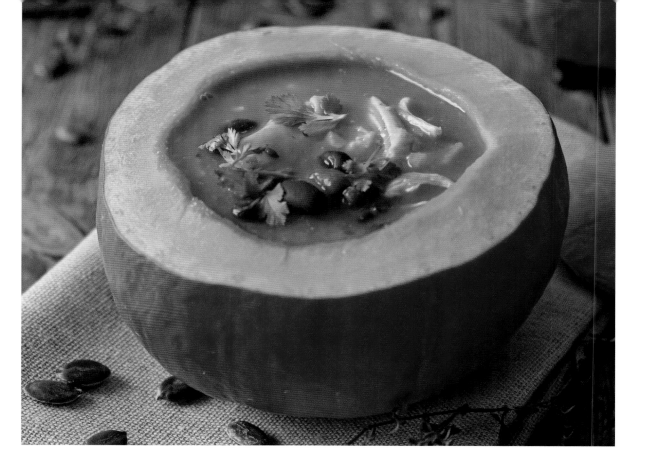

1 In a large pot, heat the oil over medium heat. Add the chicken. When slightly browned but not yet cooked through, add the onion, celery, carrot, and serrano pepper in the pot. Sauté until the onions are translucent and the chicken is cooked through. Add the garlic and continue sautéing for 1 minute, or until the garlic is fragrant.

2 Add the chicken broth and pumpkin purée, stirring to combine. Stir in the rice, black beans, cumin, and chili powder. Bring to a slow boil. Reduce the heat to medium-low and simmer for 25 to 30 minutes, or until the rice is cooked. Season with salt and pepper. Taste and adjust spiciness with extra serrano pepper and chili powder, if desired.

3 Transfer the soup into the hollowed-out pumpkins (if using) or bowls, and top with fresh parsley.

anita's tip Serving this sweet and spicy soup in hollowed out pumpkins is an adorable idea for a cozy get-together, a fall holiday party, or even Thanksgiving table! But if you're not looking to go all out, simplify it by skipping the hollowed-out pumpkins and serve in regular soup bowls.

| S, DF, GF | EASE: ●●○ | MAKES: 8 servings (groups 1 & 2) 6 servings (group 3) | TIME: 9 hours

slow-cooker shredded beef barbacoa

what you'll need:

2 lbs. (900 g) chuck roast
1 teaspoon salt
½ teaspoon ground black pepper
2 tablespoons (30 ml) plus 2 teaspoons (10 ml) extra-virgin olive oil, divided
1 cup (235 ml) low-sodium beef broth, divided
3 canned chipotle chilies, or more to taste
4 cloves garlic, minced
1 tablespoon (7 g) ground cumin
½ tablespoon (2 g) dried oregano
2 bay leaves
Juice of 2 limes

1 Cut the chuck roast into 3 to 4 pieces and trim any visible pieces of fat. Season with salt and pepper.

2 Heat 1 tablespoon (15 ml) of oil in a large, nonstick skillet over medium-high heat. Sear the roast pieces until browned on all sides. Transfer to the slow cooker in an even layer.

3 In a blender or food processor, blend together ¼ cup (60 ml) beef broth, chipotle chilies, garlic, and 1 tablespoon oil until well puréed.

4 In a medium bowl, whisk together the chipotle mixture, remaining beef broth, cumin, and oregano. Pour the mixture over beef in a slow cooker. Tuck bay leaves between beef portions.

5 Cover and cook on low heat for about 8 hours.

6 Remove the beef from the slow cooker, leaving the broth in the cooker, and shred using two forks. Stir the lime juice into broth. Return the beef to the slow cooker and cook on low for 30 minutes. Strain the liquid from beef and serve.

NOTE: *To customize into a meal, serve each serving of shredded beef barbacoa with unlimited non-starchy vegetables and:*

Group 1: 1 portion of starch
Group 2: 1 portion of fat and 1 portion of starch
Group 3: 1½ portions of fat and 1 portion of starch

anita's tip Roll up shredded beef barbacoa in a tortilla or create your own Chipotle-style barbacoa rice bowl! Although it's traditionally made with lean chuck roast, you can also use chicken breast for variety.

DINNER

| S, GF | EASE:
●●○ | MAKES:
2 servings | TIME:
20 minutes |

supreme mini pizza cups

what you'll need:

4 quick sprays cooking oil
2 (6-inch [15-cm]) tortilla wraps of
  choice
3 tablespoons (45 ml) crushed
  tomatoes
2 ounces (60 g) cooked sweet Italian
  sausage, crumbled
¼ cup (40 g) chopped red bell pepper
4 olives, sliced
2 slices red onion
3 tablespoons (15 g) shredded
  part-skim mozzarella cheese

1 Preheat the oven to 400°F (200°C). Spray a muffin pan with cooking spray.

2 Using a biscuit cutter or drinking glass, cut each tortilla wrap into rounds. Fit each round down into each muffin cup.

3 Place a 1 teaspoon of crushed tomatoes in the bottom of each cup. Sprinkle sausage, bell peppers, onions, and olives in each cup. Then, top each cup with shredded mozzarella.

4 Bake in the oven for 8 to 12 minutes, or until the cheese is melted and tortilla rounds are crispy. Remove and cool before using a fork to transfer mini pizza cups from the muffin pan to serve.

DF, V, V+: *To make this recipe dairy-free, swap mozzarella for plant-based mozzarella-style shreds. To make it plant-based, swap Italian sausage for meatless crumbles.*

anita's tip Apart from being the perfect snack, these mini pizza cups make such fun finger food—perfect for get-togethers and parties with friends!

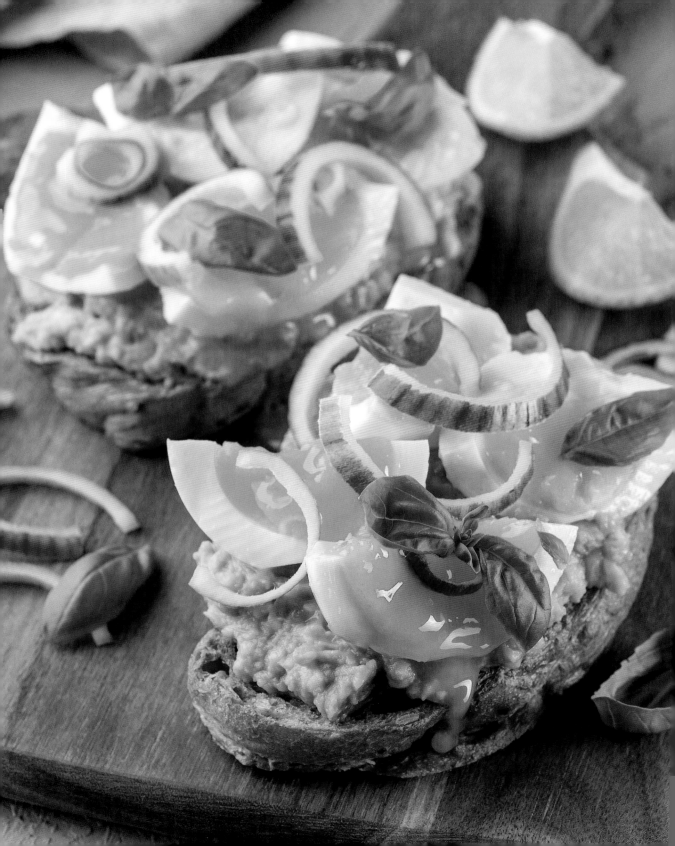

S, DF, GF, V

EASE:
●●○

MAKES:
1 serving

TIME:
15 minutes

sunny-side egg avo toast

what you'll need:

1 slice bread of choice
1 small egg
¼ small avocado
Juice of ½ lime
Dash of salt and pepper
2 rings sliced red onion
Fresh basil leaves, optional

1   Toast the bread in a toaster or in a small, nonstick pan over medium-high heat until crisp and golden on both sides.

2   While toasting the bread, bring a medium pot of water to a boil over high heat. Reduce the heat to medium, so the water maintains a gentle boil. Carefully lower the egg into the water and cook for 7 minutes. Make sure you don't cook the egg any longer than that unless you want it hard boiled.

3   While the egg is boiling, fill a bowl with cold water and ice. Remove the egg from the hot water using a slotted spoon, and immediately add it to the ice bath. Allow to chill for at least 3 minutes before peeling.

4   Meanwhile, mash the avocado with a fork and add the lime juice. Spoon the mashed avocado over the toast. Cut the egg and place it on top of the toast. Sprinkle with salt and pepper, and serve with sliced red onion and basil, if using.

anita's tip To make this toast suitable for vegans, swap out the egg for any plant-based protein from the food swap list (page 64). Alternatively, you can make it a traditional avocado toast with sliced tomato on top and roll over the protein portion for another meal in the day.

AM SNACKS

| S, DF, GF | EASE: ●○○ | MAKES: 2 servings | TIME: 5 minutes |

tuscan tuna kidney bean salad

what you'll need:

- 2 teaspoons (10 ml) extra-virgin olive oil
- 4 ounces (115 g) solid tuna in water, drained
- 1 cup (250 g) canned red kidney beans, drained and rinsed
- 2 tablespoons (20 g) finely chopped red onion
- 1 tablespoon (15 ml) fresh lemon juice
- 1 tablespoon (3 g) finely chopped fresh basil

1 In a mixing bowl, whisk together the oil, tuna, and beans. Add the red onion and stir in the lemon juice. Toss to combine.

2 Sprinkle with fresh basil.

anita's tip Get inspired by Mediterranean flavors with a super quick snack that's so easy to take with you in a container! It'll take you less than 5 minutes to toss everything together.

AM SNACKS

S, DF, GF EASE: ●●○ MAKES: 2 servings TIME: 30 minutes

louisiana pineapple chicken foil packets

what you'll need:

5 ounces (140 g) uncooked chicken
   breast, skinless and boneless
1 teaspoon Cajun seasoning (page 84),
   or more to taste
¼ teaspoon salt
1 cup (165 g) chopped pineapple
1 tablespoon (15 ml) lime juice
¼ cup (4 g) chopped fresh cilantro

1 Prepare a grill to medium-high heat or set the oven temperature to 420°F (215°C).

2 Tear two large pieces of aluminum foil and place one on top of the other. Add the chicken in the center. Spray with cooking spray and sprinkle Cajun seasoning evenly on top. Then, sprinkle with salt. Lay the pineapple on top of the chicken.

3 Tightly seal the foil pack and place it on the grill or in the oven. Grill for about 8 to 10 minutes; if cooking in the oven, bake for about 16 to 18 minutes, or until the chicken is cooked through.

4 Let the packet rest for 5 minutes before serving. Drizzle with lime juice and cut chicken into chunks before serving. Top with fresh cilantro.

anita's tip Looking to switch up the flavors? Replace Cajun seasoning with barbecue sauce for pineapple BBQ chicken!

S, DF, GF

EASE:
●●○

MAKES:
2 servings

TIME:
10 minutes

fiery orange shrimp salad

what you'll need:

½ teaspoon dried oregano

¼ teaspoon red pepper flakes

1 teaspoon hot sauce, or more to taste

1 tablespoon (15 ml) lime juice

10 ounces (285 g) jumbo shrimp, peeled and deveined

4 quick sprays of cooking oil

¼ cup (30 g) thinly sliced red onion

1 cup (150 g) cherry tomatoes

2 small oranges, peeled and sliced into circles

¼ cup (4 g) finely chopped fresh cilantro

1   In a small bowl, combine the oregano, red pepper flakes, hot sauce, and lime juice with two tablespoons (30 ml) of water. In a separate bowl, add the shrimp and stir in half the marinade.

2   Preheat a grill or grill pan over medium heat and spray with cooking oil. Cook the marinated shrimp until it curls and turns pink, about 2 to 3 minutes per side.

3   In a salad bowl, toss the onion, cherry tomatoes, oranges, and cilantro. Drizzle with the remaining marinade. Transfer the salad to a serving platter and top with the shrimp.

anita's tip The sweetness of orange and cherry tomatoes paired with a surprising punch of heat adds a delightful summertime burst to the salad. If meal prepping, store the marinade and other ingredients separately and combine when making it, so the dish doesn't get soggy when stored.

PM SNACKS

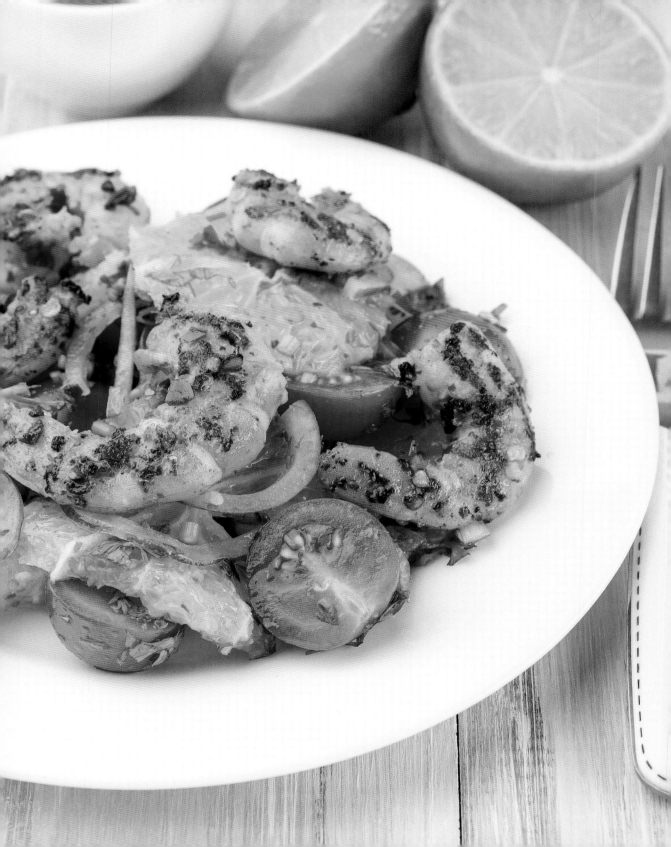

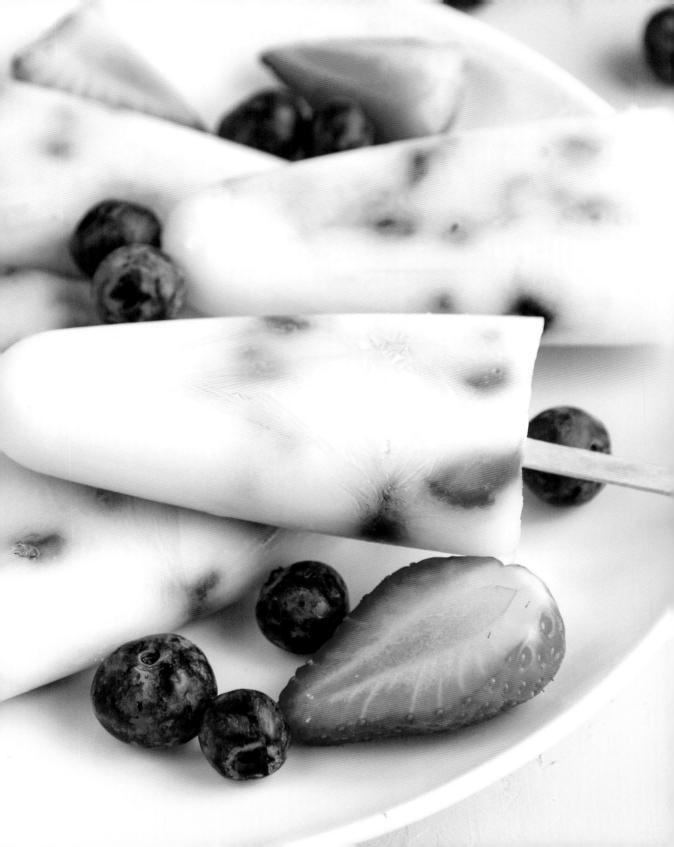

 S, GF, V

EASE:
●○○

MAKES:
2 servings

TIME:
5 hours 15 minutes

red, white & blue ice pops

what you'll need:

1 cup (170 g) mixed berries, chopped
1⅓ cups (270 g) low-fat Greek yogurt,
   vanilla or plain
2 teaspoons (15 g) honey

1 Stir together the mixed berries and yogurt until well combined.

2 Spoon the mixture into popsicle molds. Insert sticks and freeze until hard, at least 5 hours or overnight.

3 Before serving, to loosen, run the mold under warm water for a few seconds.

anita's tip The number of ice pops this recipe yields will depend on the size of your molds. The standard sizes fit about ⅓ cup of yogurt-berry mix totaling 4 ice pops, or 2 ice pops per serving.

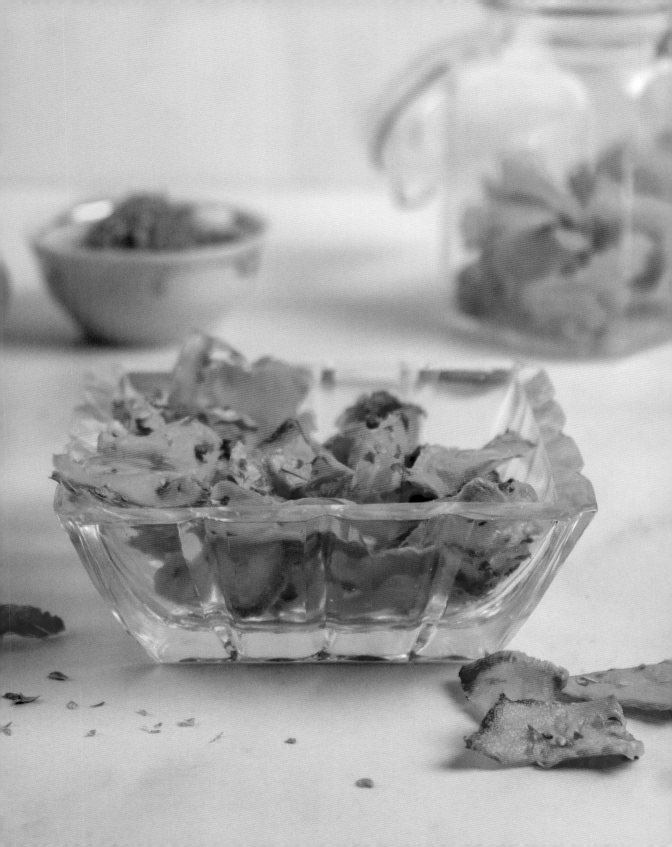

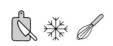

S, DF, GF, V, V+	**EASE:** ●●○	**MAKES:** 1 portion starch 1 portion fat	**TIME:** 15 minutes

air-fryer butternut squash chips

what you'll need:

7 ounces (200 g) uncooked butternut
squash
1 teaspoon extra-virgin olive oil
½ teaspoon herbes de Provence
(page 85)
Dash of salt

1 Peel the butternut squash and scoop out the seeds.

2 Starting from the neck of the butternut squash, cut it into thin (about ⅛-inch [3-mm]) chips. Try to cut the chips to equal size for even cooking. Place the chips and oil in a medium bowl. Toss to combine.

3 Air fry at 380°F (190°C) for 4 to 5 minutes. Flip the chips over and fry for 4 to 5 minutes, until they are crisp. Check the chips frequently to make sure they don't burn.

4 Remove from the air fryer, and season with herbes de Provence and salt.

anita's tip If you have a mandoline slicer or peeler, it will come handy in the slicing process to ensure that the chips are cut thin and even. Pair this with the Smoked Paprika Aioli on (page 191).

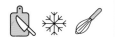
crispy air-fryer fries

what you'll need:

18 ounces (500 g) russet potatoes (about 3 small)
4 teaspoons (20 ml) extra-virgin olive oil
1 teaspoon onion powder
½ teaspoon garlic powder
¼ teaspoon dried oregano
¼ teaspoon dried basil
½ teaspoon salt
¼ teaspoon ground black pepper
2 teaspoons (5 g) smoked paprika, optional
Dash of cayenne pepper, optional

1 Peel the potatoes and slice lengthwise into ¼-inch (6-mm)-thick fries. Soak them in a bowl of water for at least 30 minutes.

2 Drain the potatoes and pat them dry. In a dry bowl, add the oil, onion powder, garlic powder, oregano, basil, salt, and pepper. Add the smoked paprika and cayenne pepper, if using. Add the potatoes and toss well using your hands.

3 Preheat your air fryer to 380°F (190°C), or per appliance instructions. Cook for 10 minutes, then toss the fries and cook for 6 to 10 minutes, or until they are golden and crispy.

anita's tip Soaking the potatoes before seasoning helps remove excess starch so the fries come out perfectly crispy on the outside yet tender on the inside.

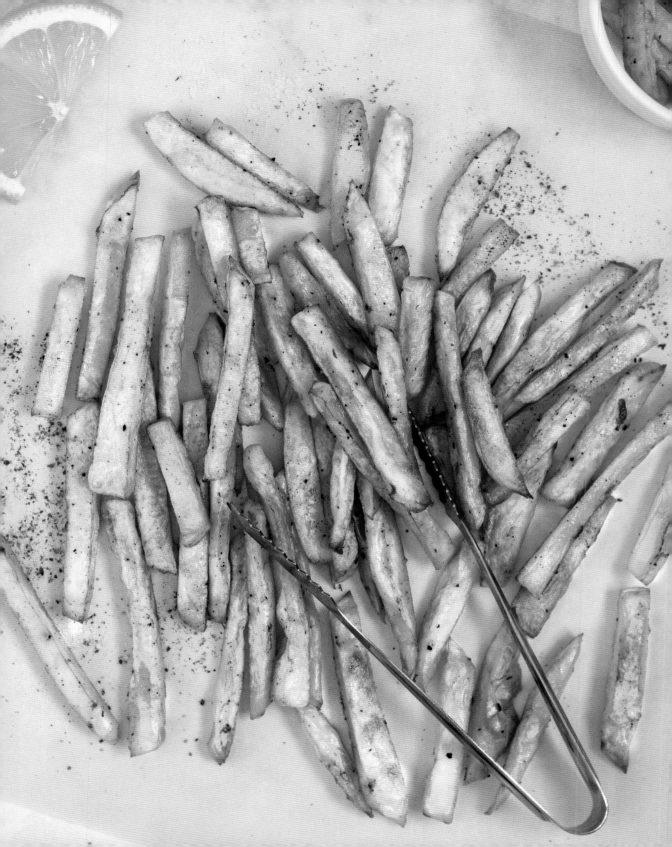

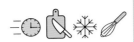 S, DF, GF, V, V+

 EASE:
●○○

 MAKES:
3 portions fruit

 TIME:
10 minutes

fruity summer salad

what you'll need:

1 cup (145 g) fresh strawberries, sliced
1 cup (175 g) diced mango
¼ cup (30 g) thinly sliced red onion
4 cups (220 g) spring mix greens
¼ teaspoon dried mint, optional

1 Mix the strawberries, mango, and red onion with the spring mix. Sprinkle with mint, if using.

anita's tip Adding fruit to a traditional green salad gives it an exciting twist. It's also a great way to get your fruit portions in! If you have rollover portions of fat, pair with Better Than Store-Bought Vinaigrette (page 193) for a lemony kick.

SIDES

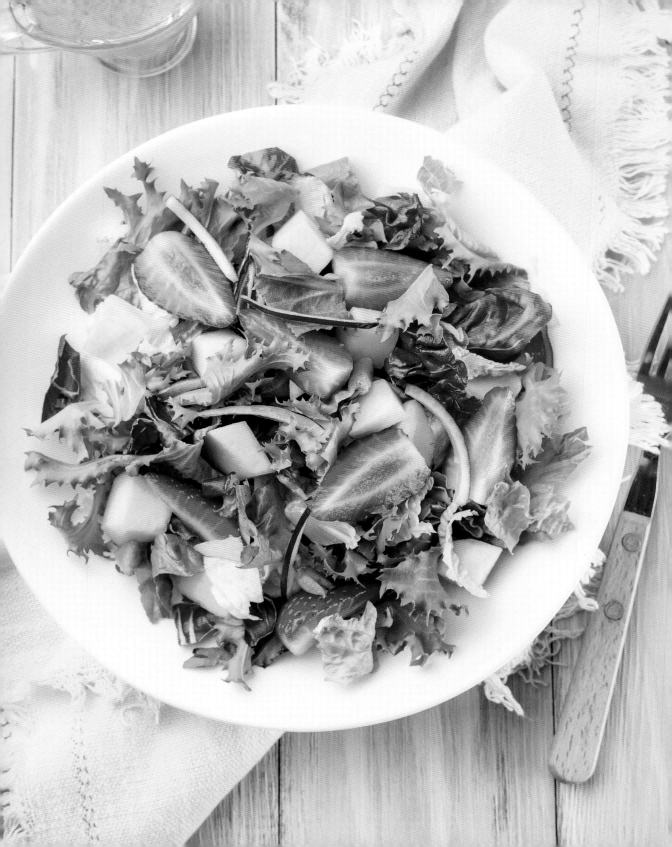

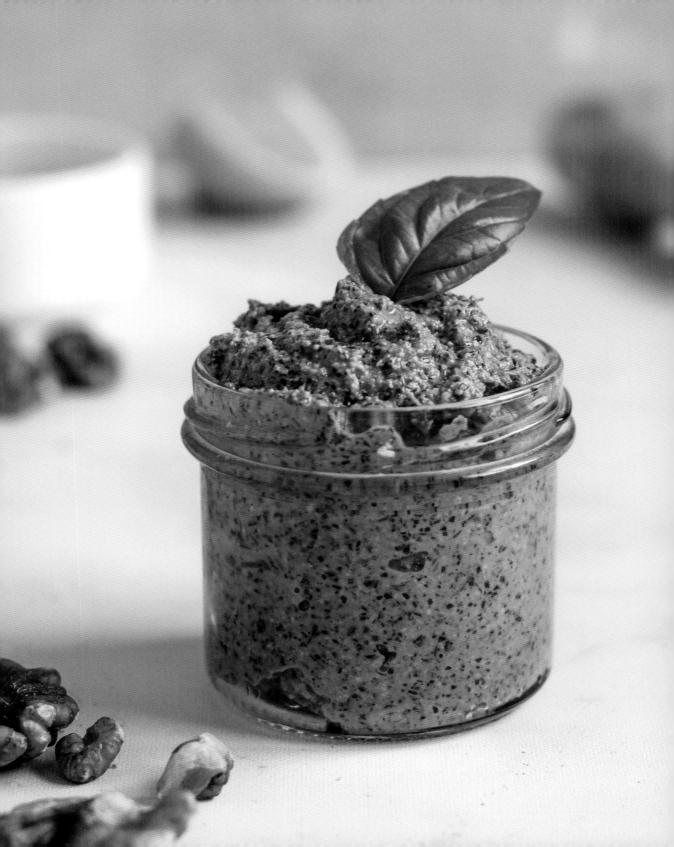

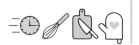 S, DF, GF, V, V+

 EASE:
●○○

MAKES:
10 portions fat

 TIME:
5 minutes

creamy blender pesto sauce

what you'll need:

1 (1.25-ounce, or 35 g) pack of fresh basil leaves

3 cloves garlic, peeled and roughly chopped

1 tablespoon (15 ml) fresh lemon juice, or more to taste

2 tablespoons (30 ml) extra-virgin olive oil

¼ cup (30 g) chopped walnuts

1 In a blender, combine the basil, garlic, lemon juice, and oil. Blend until smooth.

2 Add the walnuts and blend again until the consistency is creamy. For a lemonier pesto flavor, add extra lemon juice, to taste.

3 Store in an airtight container in the refrigerator for up to 1 week or pour into ice cube trays and freeze until needed.

anita's tip This fresh pesto sauce has been my go-to for years! It's so much better than any store-bought pesto I've tried. Toss it with chicken, shrimp, or veggie pasta, or enjoy as a spread on bread. The recipe doesn't have any added salt, allowing you to adjust it based on your salt intake for the day.

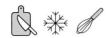

S, DF, GF, V, V+

EASE:
●○○

MAKES:
24 portions fat

TIME:
3 hours 5 minutes

mabel's chimichurri criollo

what you'll need:

½ cup (120 ml) extra-virgin olive oil
¼ cup (60 ml) red wine vinegar
¼ cup (15 g) finely minced fresh parsley
2 cloves garlic, finely minced
1 tablespoon (10 g) finely minced red chili
¼ cup (40 g) finely minced yellow onion
1 teaspoon dried oregano
½ teaspoon salt

1 In a medium bowl, mix all the ingredients together. Refrigerate in an airtight container for at least 3 hours or overnight before serving. Store in the fridge for up to 5 to 7 days.

anita's tip This is a vibrant Northern Argentinian family recipe that is traditionally brushed over grilled and baked meat dishes, but it also goes great with pork chops and chicken. To freeze, put the chimichurri sauce in an ice cube tray with a little water. Once frozen, store the cubes in a freezer bag.

SAUCES & DIPS

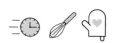

| | S, GF, V | EASE:
●○○ | MAKES:
4 portions fat | TIME:
3 minutes |

smoked paprika aioli

what you'll need:

¼ cup (60 g) low-fat mayonnaise
1 clove garlic, minced
¼ teaspoon garlic powder
1 teaspoon smoked paprika
½ teaspoon fresh lemon juice
Dash of salt

1   In a small bowl, combine the mayonnaise, garlic, garlic powder, paprika, lemon juice, and salt. Whisk until smooth.

anita's tip Everyone who's tasted this restaurant-style dip has fallen head over heels in love with it! Serve it with vegetable sticks, baked sweet potato wedges, or Crispy Air-Fryer Fries (page 184).

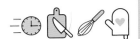 S, GF, V

 EASE:
●○○

 MAKES:
1 portion protein
1 portion fat

 TIME:
5 minutes

better than store-bought ranch

what you'll need:

⅓ cup (65 g) plain nonfat Greek yogurt
1 tablespoon (15 g) low-fat mayonnaise
¾ teaspoon garlic powder
¾ teaspoon onion powder
½ teaspoon dried parsley
½ teaspoon dried chives
¼ teaspoon dried dill
¼ teaspoon salt
⅛ teaspoon ground black pepper
½ teaspoon fresh lemon juice
½ teaspoon Dijon mustard

1 Combine the yogurt, mayonnaise, garlic powder, onion powder, parsley, chives, dill, salt, pepper, lemon juice, and Dijon mustard in a small bowl. Mix well to combine. Refrigerate in an airtight container for up to 5 days.

anita's tip You'd be surprised to find how easy it is to make ranch sauce at home! Enjoy it as a dip or dressing, or to toss depending on the recipe. It goes great with veggie sticks.

SAUCES & DIPS

S, DF, GF, V

EASE:
●○○

MAKES:
12 portions fat

TIME:
5 minutes

better than store-bought vinaigrette

what you'll need:

¼ cup (60 ml) fresh lemon juice
1 clove garlic, minced
1 teaspoon Dijon mustard
¼ teaspoon salt
⅛ teaspoon ground black pepper
½ teaspoon honey
¼ cup (60 ml) extra-virgin olive oil

1 In a small bowl, whisk together the lemon juice, garlic, mustard, salt, pepper, and honey. Drizzle in the olive oil while whisking and continue to mix until the dressing is emulsified.

anita's tip You can store this delicious lemon-honey vinaigrette dressing in the fridge for up to 1 week. When you take it out let sit at room temperature to soften for a few minutes before using.

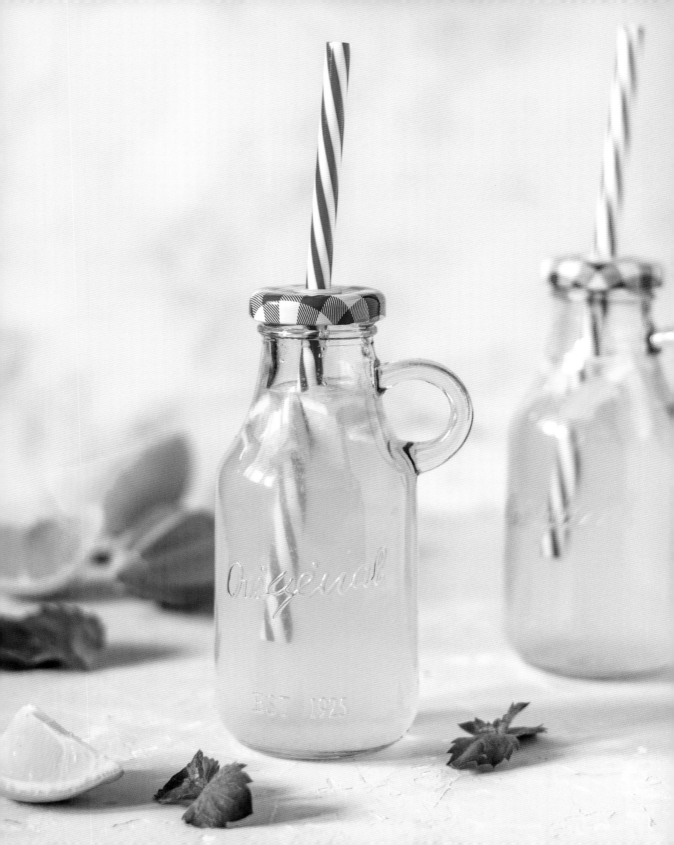

S, DF, GF, V, V+

EASE:
●○○

MAKES:
4 servings

TIME:
5 minutes

homemade old-fashioned lemonade

what you'll need:

Juice of 3 large lemons
1 teaspoon dry stevia, or more to taste
Ice, optional
Mint, optional for garnish

1   Mix all lemon juice, 1 quart (about 1 L) of water, and stevia together. Store in a pitcher. Serve cold and if desired, over ice.

> **anita's tip** Lemonade can help you bump up your water intake, especially on hot summer days! Best of all, this lemonade recipe is untracked and won't count toward your meals.

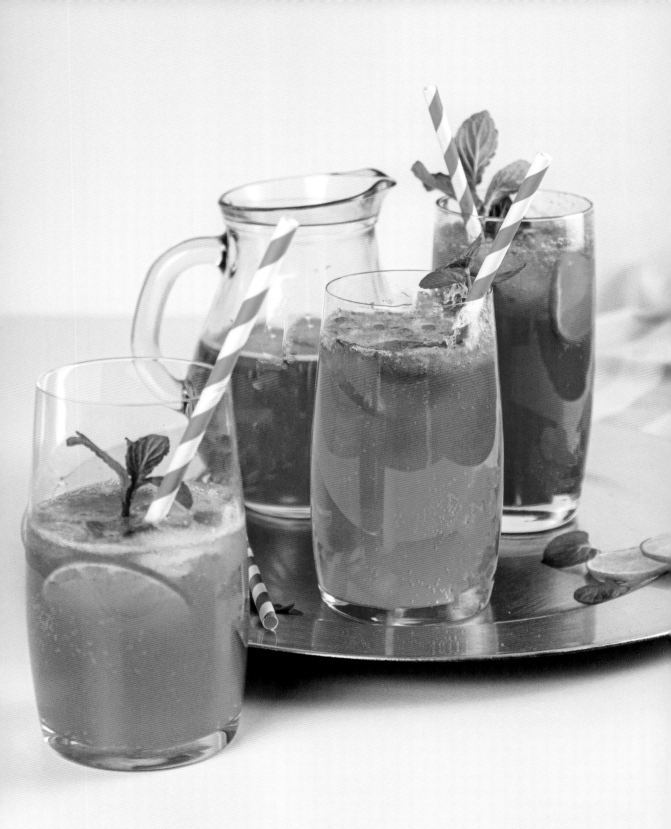

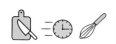

S, DF, GF, V, V+

EASE:
●○○

MAKES:
3 portions fruit

TIME:
5 minutes

bubbly watermelon mint mocktails

what you'll need:

3 cups (450 g) cubed seedless
   watermelon
Juice of 2 limes
5–6 fresh mint leaves, or more to taste
Ice cubes
2 cups (475 ml) sparkling water

1   Place the watermelon into a blender with the lime juice and mint leaves. Blend until smooth. To remove pulp, pour through a strainer.

2   Fill 3 tall glasses with ice. Pour in the watermelon juice until each glass is halfway full. Top with sparkling water. Gently stir the drinks with a spoon and enjoy.

anita's tip This fizzy summer day staple will bring a carefree beach vibe to your home! Choose seedless watermelon, which makes this recipe much easier and quicker.

TREATS

S, DF, GF, V, V+

EASE:
●●○

MAKES:
2 portions starch

TIME:
1 hour

arroz con leche rice pudding

what you'll need:

2 ounces (60 g) uncooked long-grain brown rice

2 cups (475 ml) unsweetened almond milk, divided

1 tablespoon (8 g) dry stevia, or more to taste

Pinch of salt

½ teaspoon pure vanilla extract

½ teaspoon ground cinnamon, plus more for garnish

1 Rinse the brown rice under cold water in a fine-mesh strainer for 2 to 3 minutes. Drain.

2 In a small pot, combine 1 cup (235 ml) of almond milk, the stevia, salt, vanilla, and drained brown rice. Bring to a boil over medium-high heat.

3 Turn the heat down to low and cover the pot with lid. Let simmer for about 30 to 35 minutes, stirring occasionally.

4 Add ½ cup (120 ml) of almond milk and let simmer for 10 to 15 minutes, or until the rice is soft and chewy. Add more stevia or cinnamon, if desired.

5 When cooled, store in an airtight container for up to 3 to 4 days in the fridge. Stir in the remaining ¼ cup (60 ml) of almond milk per serving before eating, and sprinkle with cinnamon.

anita's tip Sugar is replaced with the natural sweetness of stevia in this take on a classic rice pudding. A little goes a long way, which makes tasting essential while making any recipe that's sweetened by stevia!

TREATS

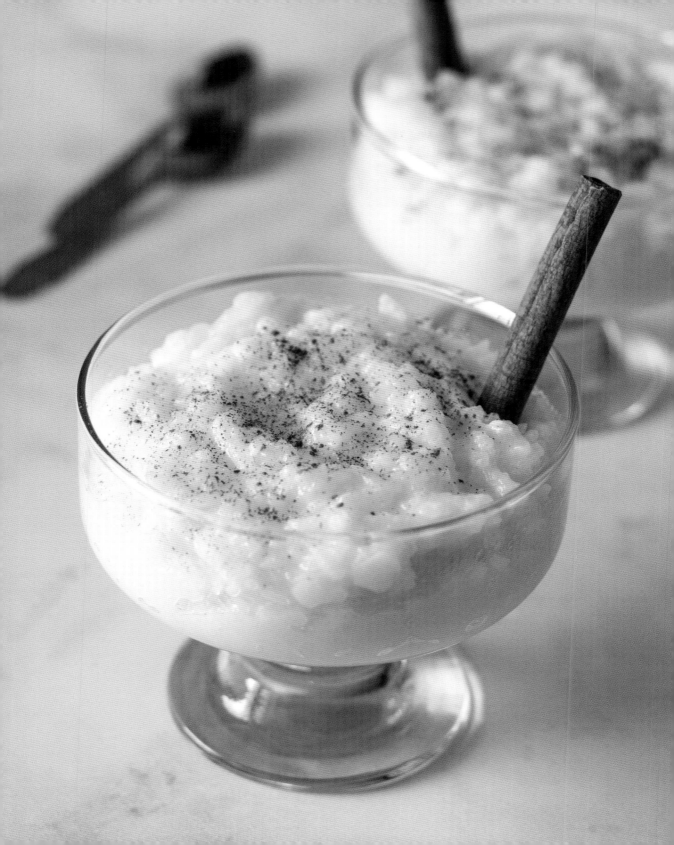

S, DF, GF, V

EASE:
●○○

MAKES:
8 servings

TIME:
20 minutes

coquito coconut drops

What you'll need:

1 cup (85 g) shredded unsweetened
    coconut
1 small egg
1½ teaspoons dry stevia
½ teaspoon pure vanilla extract
½ teaspoon baking powder

1 Preheat the oven to 350°F (175°C).

2 In a small mixing bowl, combine coconut, egg, stevia, vanilla, and baking powder. Divide the mixture into 8 small pieces and pinch each one into a cone-like shape using your hands. Place them on a baking dish.

3 Bake for about 15 minutes, or until the top of the coconut drops start turning golden brown.

anita's tip Coquitos are the sweetest way to enjoy fat portions in the form of mini desserts! Each drop counts as 1 portion.

TREATS

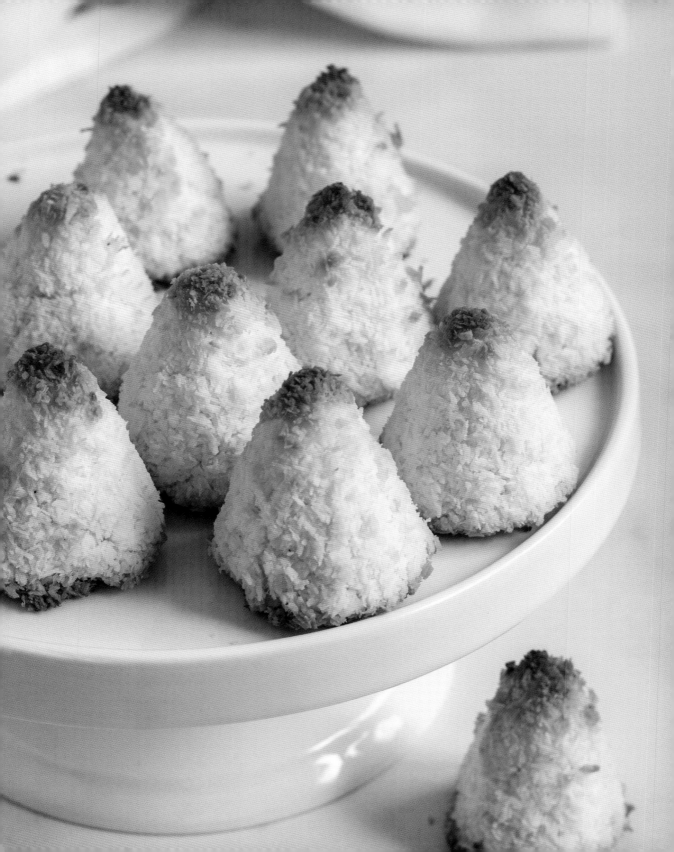

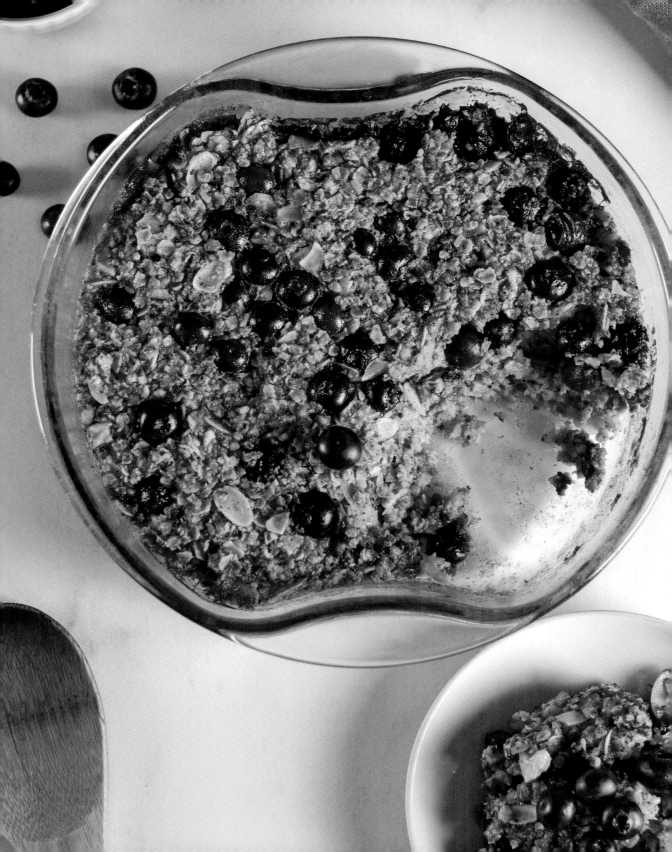

S, GF, V

EASE:
● ● ○

MAKES:
6 servings

TIME:
35 minutes

blueberry baked oat bars

what you'll need:

3 tablespoons (40 g) unsalted butter, softened, divided

2 small ripe bananas, mashed

1 cup (155 g) frozen blueberries

2 cups (190 g) old-fashioned rolled oats

1 small egg

2 tablespoons (40 g) maple syrup

1 teaspoon pure vanilla extract

1 teaspoon baking powder

½ teaspoon ground cinnamon

⅛ teaspoon salt

1 Preheat the oven to 375°F (190°C).

2 In a medium bowl, combine 2 tablespoons (30 g) of butter, bananas, frozen blueberries, oats, egg, maple syrup, vanilla, baking powder, cinnamon, and salt. Mix well.

3 Grease an 8- x 8-inch (20- x 20-cm) baking dish with the remaining butter. Transfer mixture to the dish.

4 Place in the oven and bake until the center is set, about 30 minutes. Remove from the oven and let cool for a few minutes. Cut into 6 equal bars. Serve warm or cooled.

anita's tip To make it the ultimate sweet treat, place a can of unsweetened coconut cream in the fridge overnight. Store the liquid part for use another time and whip the solid cream with a handheld mixer. Taste and add a dash of vanilla extract and stevia as needed. One tablespoon counts as a portion of fat, which you can borrow from another meal! Each serving of this recipe counts as 1 portion starch, 1 portion of fruit, and 1 portion of fat.

TREATS

about the author

Anita Rincón is an author, speaker, and founder of global women's wellness company Sculpt. Born in Finland and spending her childhood and adolescence in Europe and South America, Anita took a leap to follow her dreams by moving to the United States in her early twenties. Since then, she has worked tirelessly toward her mission of making wellness accessible and inclusive to everyone. She holds a master's degree in nutrition science with a focus on obesity and weight management. Together with leading nutrition, fitness, and wellness professionals, Anita provides evidence-based, holistic solutions to empower and inspire women around the world to transform their lives through Sculpt's online platforms, mobile app, product lines, streaming series, podcast, and events. Anita lives in New York City, and her extraordinary story has been celebrated by Forbes, Cosmopolitan, NBC, and Telemundo, among other news outlets. In her spare time, Anita enjoys volunteering at local animal shelters and has two rescue pets of her own.

Connect with Anita: ☐ thesculptplan.com   ⬡ @sculptonline

references

Martin CB, Herrick KA, Sarafrazi N, Ogden CL. Attempts to lose weight among adults in the United States, 2013-2016. *NCHS Data Brief*. 2018;(313):1-8.

Wing RR, Phelan S. Long-term weight loss maintenance. *Am J Clin Nutr*. 2005;82(1 Suppl):222S-225S. doi:10.1093/ajcn/82.1.222S

Almiron-Roig E, Solis-Trapala I, Dodd J, Jebb SA. Estimating food portions. Influence of unit number, meal type and energy density. *Appetite*. 2013;71:95-103. doi:10.1016/j.appet.2013.07.012

McPherson R. Genetic contributors to obesity. *Can J Cardiol*. 2007;23 Suppl A(Suppl A):23A-27A. doi:10.1016/s0828-282x(07)71002-4

Nedeltcheva AV, Kilkus JM, Imperial J, Schoeller DA, Penev PD. Insufficient sleep undermines dietary efforts to reduce adiposity. *Ann Intern Med*. 2010;153(7):435-441. doi:10.7326/0003-4819-153-7-201010050-00006

Urban LE, Weber JL, Heyman MB, et al. Energy contents of frequently ordered restaurant meals and comparison with human energy requirements and U.S. Department of Agriculture database information: a multisite randomized study. *J Acad Nutr Diet*. 2016;116(4):590-8. e6. doi:10.1016/j.jand.2015.11.009

Ingels JS, Misra R, Stewart J, Lucke-Wold B, Shawley-Brzoska S. The effect of adherence to dietary tracking on weight loss: using HLM to model weight loss over time. *J Diabetes Res*. 2017;2017:6951495. doi:10.1155/2017/6951495

Zheng Y, Klem ML, Sereika SM, Danford CA, Ewing LJ, Burke LE. Self-weighing in weight management: a systematic literature review. *Obesity (Silver Spring)*. 2015;23(2):256-265. doi:10.1002/oby.20946

Painter SL, Ahmed R, Hill JO, et al. What matters in weight loss? An in-depth analysis of self-monitoring. *J Med Internet Res*. 2017;19(5):e160. doi:10.2196/jmir.7457

Olivier M, López-Santiago R, Contreras I. Chronic intake of commercial sweeteners induces changes in feeding behavior and signaling pathways related to the control of appetite in BALB/c mice. *Biomed Res Int*. 2018;2018:3628121. doi:10.1155/2018/3628121

Hetherington MM, Blundell-Birtill P, Caton SJ, et al. Understanding the science of portion control and the art of downsizing. *Proc Nutr Soc*. 2018;77(3):347-355. doi:10.1017/S0029665118000435

Van der Valk ES, Savas M, van Rossum EFC. Stress and obesity: are there more susceptible individuals? *Curr Obes Rep*. 2018;7(2):193-203. doi:10.1007/s13679-018-0306-y

Basso JC, Suzuki WA. The effects of acute exercise on mood, cognition, neurophysiology, and neurochemical pathways: a review. *Brain Plast*. 2017;2(2):127-152. doi:10.3233/BPL-160040

Grandner MA. The cost of sleep lost: implications for health, performance, and the bottom line. *Am J Health Promot*. 2018;32(7):1629-1634. doi:10.1177/0890117118790621a

Knutson KL, Van Cauter E. Associations between sleep loss and increased risk of obesity and diabetes. *Ann N Y Acad Sci*. 2008;1129:287-304. doi:10.1196/annals.1417.033

Calvin AD, Carter RE, Adachi T, et al. Effects of experimental sleep restriction on caloric intake and activity energy expenditure. *Chest*. 2013;144(1):79-86. doi:10.1378/chest.12-2829

Taheri S, Lin L, Austin D, Young T, Mignot E. Short sleep duration is associated with reduced leptin, elevated ghrelin, and increased body mass index. *PLoS Med*. 2004;1(3):e62. doi:10.1371/journal.pmed.0010062

Yau YH, Potenza MN. Stress and eating behaviors. *Minerva Endocrinol*. 2013;38(3):255-267.

Ma X, Yue ZQ, Gong ZQ, et al. The effect of diaphragmatic breathing on attention, negative affect and stress in healthy adults. *Front Psychol*. 2017;8:874. doi:10.3389/fpsyg.2017.00874

Warren JM, Smith N, Ashwell M. A structured literature review on the role of mindfulness, mindful eating and intuitive eating in changing eating behaviours: effectiveness and associated potential mechanisms. *Nutr Res Rev*. 2017;30(2):272-283. doi:10.1017/S0954422417000154

Eom H, Lee D, Cho Y, Moon J. The association between meal regularity and weight loss among women in commercial weight loss programs. *Nutr Res Pract*. 2022;16(2):205-216. doi:10.4162/nrp.2022.16.2.205

index